MW01382616

Medicode's 2000 Publications & Software For Coders

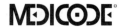

Medicode, 5225 Wiley Post Way, Suite 500, Salt Lake City, UT 84116 • 801.536.1000 • FAX 801.536.1011

ORDER TOLL FREE OR CALL FOR A FREE CATALOG 800.999.4600
AVAILABLE FROM YOUR MEDICAL BOOKSTORE OR DISTRIBUTOR.

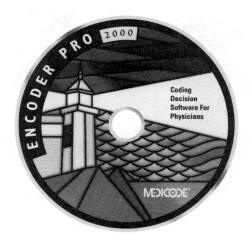

It's Easy to Tap into the Power of *Encoder Pro*

Encoder Pro
(Item #2717)   **$499⁹⁵**

Quickly look up ICD-9-CM, CPT and HCPCS Level II codes with the fastest, easiest and most powerful physician coding software available. Access Medicode's database of top selling publications instantaneously, to ensure all your claims are properly coded. See for yourself the advantages this invaluable resource will bring to your office:

- **NEW! View Index Results.** Instantaneously search ICD-9, CPT, and HCPCS indexes.
- **NEW! View CPT Assistant References.** See which editions of *CPT Assistant* have articles relating to CPT codes.
- **NEW! Alerts for deleted codes.** Deleted code alerts are displayed if a code is no longer valid. Provides cross-reference to valid codes where applicable.
- **NEW! Revised and New Code Icons.** New icons for ICD-9, CPT, and HCPCS Level II codes identify revised and new codes.
- **Easy to Use.** Using *Encoder Pro* is intuitive. Accessing information is just a click away.
- **Find the Right Code Fast.** *Encoder Pro's* powerful search engine guides you to the right code.
- **Save Time.** Search results display instantaneously. No more thumbing through various code books.
- **Interface Capability.** Active X technology allows *Encoder Pro* to be interfaced with practice management software.
- **HCFA-1500.** Enter claim information into electronic form. Save and or print.
- **Windows™ Compatible.** Copy codes and descriptions and reference information to the Windows clipboard for use in other Windows applications.

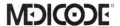

Medicode, 5225 Wiley Post Way, Suite 400, Salt Lake City, UT 84116 • 801.536.1000 • FAX 801.536.1011

ORDER TOLL FREE OR CALL FOR A FREE CATALOG 800.999.4600
AVAILABLE FROM YOUR MEDICAL BOOKSTORE OR DISTRIBUTOR.

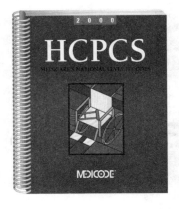

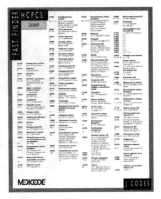

Capture Your Costs with *HCPCS* Codes

2000 HCPCS
ISBN 1-56337-301-7

(Item #2798) $49.95
Available December 1999

HCPCS ASCII File*

(Item #3906) $229.95
Available January 2000

This best-selling *HCPCS* book has many features to help you bill DME, pharmaceuticals, and select medical services easily and more accurately.

- **EXCLUSIVE! Payers Appendix.** We let you know which payers accept HCPCS Level II codes so you can file claims with confidence.

- **EXCLUSIVE! Flagged Quantity Codes.** Codes that require quantities are flagged to remind you to fill in the quantity when completing reimbursement forms.

- **EXCLUSIVE! Color tabs.** Color-coded index tabbing makes it easy to find the correct code quickly.

- **Expanded Index.** Helps you code accurately. We link brand name DME, like wheelchairs, diabetes supplies, and ostomy equipment, to their correct codes.

- **Color Coded Icons.** Codes with special Medicare instructions and coverage issues are flagged to curb claim denials.

Quick Reference Coding

2000 HCPCS Fast Finders
$24.95 per sheet
    Drug Codes (HCPCS) (Item #3129)
    Orthotics (Item #3172)
    Prosthetics (Item #3173)
    Home Health (Item #3171)
    Vision and Hearing (Item #3174)
    Physician Office Supplies (Item #3175)

Our *HCPCS Fast Finder* gives you the ability to quickly find the code that you need from among a list of more than 300 of the most commonly used codes. Each double-sided and laminated *Fast Finder* is durable, portable, and easy-to-use. Choose the one that best suits your specialty

- **Upated for 2000.** Provides current codes so that you have the most accurate information.

- **Easy-to-Use.** Lists more than 300 commonly used codes in one location.

- **Accurate.** All codes are valid and coded to the highest level of specificity.

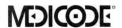

Medicode, 5225 Wiley Post Way, Suite 500, Salt Lake City, UT 84116 • 801.536.1000 • FAX 801.536.1011

ORDER TOLL FREE OR CALL FOR A FREE CATALOG 800.999.4600
AVAILABLE FROM YOUR MEDICAL BOOKSTORE OR DISTRIBUTOR.

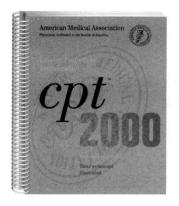

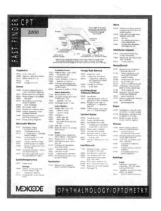

Don't Risk Filing with Obsolete CPT™ Codes

Available November 1999

Hundreds of CPT code changes will soon be in effect. Make sure you have a current CPT code book in your office — or risk rejected claims, delayed payments, and even charges of fraud and abuse!

CPT Professional Binder Version
Binder offers flexibility, color keys and illustrations.
ISBN 1-57947-019-X
(Item #2516) **$74.95**

CPT Professional Spiralbound Version
Durable and easy-to-use with color coding and illustrations.
ISBN 1-57947-018-1
(Item #2515) **$66.95**

CPT Standard Spiralbound
Economical, easy-to-use and durable
ISBN 1-57947-017-3
(Item #2518) **$51.95**

CPT Standard Softbound
AMA's economical classic
ISBN 1-57947-016-5
(Item #2517) **$47.95**

Medicodes Relative Values & CPT ASCII File*
(Item #3902) **$249.95**
Available January 2000

2000 CPT Minibooks
You can now order AMA Minibooks individually. Eight specialties to choose from for just **$29.95**

Dermatology, Plastic & Reconstructive Surgery
ISBN 1-57947-020-3
(Item #3267)

General Surgery
ISBN 1-57947-021-1
(Item #3264)

Gynecology, Obstetrics & Urology
ISBN 1-57947-022-X
(Item #3261)

Head & Neck Surgery, Oral & Maxillofacial Surgery, Ophthalmology & Otorhinolaryngology
ISBN 1-57947-023-8
(Item #3265)

Medical Specialties
ISBN 1-57947-024-6
(Item #3266)

Neurological & Orthopaedic Surgery
ISBN 1-57947-025-4
(Item #3262)

Pathology & Laboratory Medicine
ISBN 1-57947-026-2
(Item #3260)

Radiology
ISBN 1-57947-027-0
(Item #3263)

Shortcuts to Precision Coding

2000 CPT Specialty Fast Finders
Available November 1999

Each double-sided, laminated sheet provides a quick reference list of the most common CPT codes for each specialty.

- **NEW! Updated for 2000.** Prevents use of invalid codes. Only current codes are included.
- **Specialized and complete.** Includes 21 specialties on separate and laminated sheets.
- **Quick-Reference to CPT descriptions.** Condenses CPT descriptions in a format that ensures accurate coding.
- **All-inclusive code sets.** Covers the spectrum of CPT, including surgery, laboratory, radiology, medicine, E/M, and anesthesia.

$24.95 per sheet

Allergy and Immunology (Item #3150)
Cardiology (Item #3151)
Cardiovascular and Thoracic Surgery (Item #3152)
Dental/OMS (Item #3153)
Dermatology (Item #3154)
ENT (Item #3155)
Gastroenterology (Item #3156)
General Surgery (Item #3157)
Hematology/Oncology (Item #3158)
Laboratory and Pathology (Item #3159)
Neurology (Item #3160)
Obstetrics, Gynecology and Infertility (Item #3161)
Ophthalmology (Item #3162)
Orthopaedic Surgery (Item #3163)
Pediatrics (Item #3164)
Physical Medicine/Rehab/PT (Item #3165)
Plastic and Reconstructive Surgery (Item #3166)
Primary Care and Internal Medicine (Item #3167)
Psychiatry (Item #3168)
Radiology (Item #3169)
Urology and Nephrology (Item #3170)

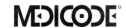

Medicode, 5225 Wiley Post Way, Suite 500, Salt Lake City, UT 84116 • 801.536.1000 • FAX 801.536.1011

ORDER TOLL FREE OR CALL FOR A FREE CATALOG 800.999.4600
AVAILABLE FROM YOUR MEDICAL BOOKSTORE OR DISTRIBUTOR.

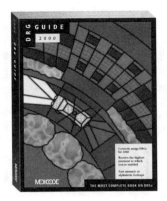

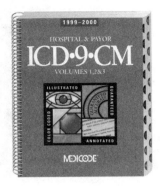

Manage Your DRG Selection Process

2000 DRG Guide
ISBN 1-56337-307-6

(Item #2530) $89⁹⁵
Available October 1999

Assigning correct DRGs is now easier than ever with *2000 DRG Guide*. This invaluable reference not only provides DRG information, but also contains DRG selection tips. All of the information you need is in one complete source.

- **EXCLUSIVE! DRG Information and Selection Tips.** Make sure you are assigning the correct DRG and receiving the highest payment to which you're entitled.
- **Indexes ICD-9-CM Codes.** Lists diagnoses and procedures numerically and alphabetically for fast lookup.
- **HCFA Rate Structure.** Identifies current relative weight, geometric mean length of stay, and average mean length of stay for each DRG.
- **DRG Drug List.** Alphabetically names brand and generic drugs that may be prescribed for conditions considered a CC.
- **DRG Decision Trees.** Easily select DRGs through flow chart type decision trees.

The Only Spiral Bound Hospital ICD-9-CM Available

1999-2000 Hospital & Payer ICD-9-CM
ISBN 1-56337-286-X

(Item #2924) $89⁹⁵
Available September 1999

ASCII File*

(Item #3900) $279⁹⁵
Available September 1999

This easy-to-use *ICD-9-CM* code book for hospitals and payers contains many valuable features to help you code accurately—all at a competitive price.

- **EXCLUSIVE! Note Saver System.** Space to write and a system to save important coding notes for next year's edition.
- **125+ Color Illustrations.** Anatomical differences are highlighted and coding issues explained.
- **2000+ Annotations.** Concise definitions aid in code selection.
- **Color Coded Tabular and Index.** Alerts coders to coding and reimbursement issues based on Medicare edits.
- **Highlighted Fourth and Fifth Digits.** Saves you from searching for the additional digit.
- **Flags Complications and Comorbidity.** Lets you know if a diagnosis could affect DRG selection.
- **AHA Coding Clinic References.** Listed next to codes to quickly find official guidelines.
- **ASCII File.** Includes ICD-9, Volumes 1 and 3 codes. Full, long, and short descriptions.

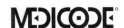

Medicode, 5225 Wiley Post Way, Suite 500, Salt Lake City, UT 84116 • 801.536.1000 • FAX 801.536.1011

ORDER TOLL FREE OR CALL FOR A FREE CATALOG 800.999.4600
AVAILABLE FROM YOUR MEDICAL BOOKSTORE OR DISTRIBUTOR.

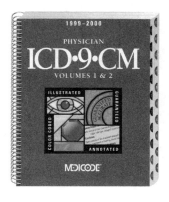

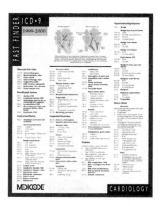

The Best Features at the Best Prices

1999-2000 Deluxe Physician ICD-9-CM
Thumb tabs, spiral binding, free ICD-9 Fast Finder
ISBN 1-56337-314-9

(Item #2709) **$69.95**
Available August 1999

1999-2000 Compact Physician ICD-9-CM
Thumb tabs, convenient size
ISBN 1-56337-313-0

(Item #2708) **$59.95**
Available August 1999

1999-2000 Standard Physician ICD-9-CM
Medicode's economical classic
ISBN 1-56337-312-2

(Item #2687) **$51.95**
Available August 1999

Medicode's *ICD-9-CM* code books offer many features at a fantastic price. Varying editions of our code books are available to keep coders accurate and meet your specific needs.

- **EXCLUSIVE! Medicare Edits.** Large scopes of non-specific codes are identified and serve as guidelines for coding and audits.
- **Color Coded.** Tabular section and icons in the index are color coded to help you code quickly and easily.
- **Illustrations and Annotations.** Helps you code accurately.
- **Fourth and Fifth Digits.** Highlighted to help you find the additional digit.

Save Time and Money

1999-2000 ICD-9 Fast Finder
Available August 1999

Each double-sided, laminated *Fast Finder* contains more than 300 diagnosis codes based on actual frequencies for 20 specialties.

- **Accurate.** All codes are valid and coded to the highest level of specificity.
- **Specific Diagnoses.** We provide more than the .89 and .99 "dump" codes.
- **Secondary Diagnoses.** Included with each specialty to provide a complete coding resource.
- **Clinically and Statistically Sound.** Provides accurate, appropriate, and comprehensive code sets developed by clinical and records specialists.

$24.95 per sheet
Allergy/Immunology (Item #3120)
Cardiology (Item #3121)
Cardiovascular/Thoracic Surgery (Item #3122)
Dental/OMS (Item #3123)
Dermatology (Item #3124)
ENT (Item #3125)
Gastroenterology (Item #3126)
General Surgery (Item #3127)
Hematology/Oncology (Item #3128)
Neurology/Oncology (Item #3130)
Ob/Gyn (Item #3131)
Ophthalmology/Optometry (Item #3132)
Orthopedics (Item #3133)
Pediatrics (Item #3134)
Physical Medicine/Rehabilitation (Item #3135)
Plastic/Reconstructive Surgery (Item #3136)
Primary Care/Internal Medicine (Item #3137)
Psychiatry (Item #3138)
Urology/Nephrology (Item #3139)

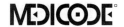

Medicode, 5225 Wiley Post Way, Suite 500, Salt Lake City, UT 84116 • 801.536.1000 • FAX 801.536.1011

ORDER TOLL FREE OR CALL FOR A FREE CATALOG 800.999.4600
AVAILABLE FROM YOUR MEDICAL BOOKSTORE OR DISTRIBUTOR.

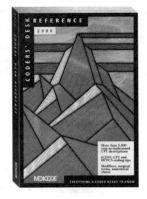

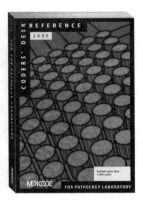

Get Instant Answers to Your Tough Coding Questions

2000 Coders' Desk Reference
ISBN 1-56337-324-6

(Item #2749) **$99.95**
Available December 1999

No matter how much experience you have using ICD-9, CPT, and HCPCS codes, there are always tough questions that hold up the billing process. And because billing errors can result in fines, you can't afford to guess. Now you can get easy-to-understand answers to your coding questions, without leaving your desk, with the *2000 Coders' Desk Reference*.

- **NEW! Improved explanations for surgical procedures.** Helps coders more accurately understand and determine CPT codes.
- **NEW! ICD-10-CM and ICD-10-PCS information.** Helps prepare for implementation in 2001.
- **NEW! 2000 CPT explanations.** CPT explanations are updated.
- **NEW! Extensive Glossary of Abbreviations, Acronyms, and Symbols**—now with cross-references to applicable CPT codes. Understand what the abbreviations, acronyms, and symbols mean and find out the CPT codes that use them.
- **Eponyms defined and linked.** Eponyms are cross-referenced to CPT codes.
- **Syndromes defined and coded.** Understand more than 1,000 syndromes explained and cross-referenced to *ICD-9-CM*.
- **Visual Help.** Find the right body area or incision length using the anatomical and metric conversion charts.
- **Anesthesia Crosswalk.** Outlines applicable anesthesia codes for CPT surgical procedures.

Get Fast Answers to Your Path/Lab Coding Questions

2000 Coders' Desk Reference for Pathology and Laboratory Services
ISBN 1-56337-334-3

(Item #5855) **$99.95**
Available February 2000

Code pathology and laboratory services right the first time. Increased scrutiny on path/lab claims can mean costly delays and denials... or worse. Having a resource dedicated to path/lab coding at your fingertips is essential.

The new *2000 Coders' Desk Reference for Pathology and Laboratory* gives you a wealth of information to answer your tough coding questions. You'll code more accurately, quickly, and confidently.

- **Easy-to-understand explanations of path/lab procedures.** Helps you quickly determine the appropriate CPT code.
- **Coding comments for hundreds of procedures.** Points you to more specific codes or other procedures that could apply, enabling you to code more accurately.
- **CLIA and HIPAA compliance information including detailed information on what constitutes fraud and abuse.** You can be confident that you are coding by the rules.

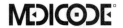

Medicode, 5225 Wiley Post Way, Suite 500, Salt Lake City, UT 84116 • 801.536.1000 • FAX 801.536.1011

ORDER TOLL FREE OR CALL FOR A FREE CATALOG 800.999.4600

AVAILABLE FROM YOUR MEDICAL BOOKSTORE OR DISTRIBUTOR.

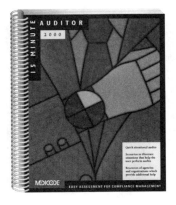

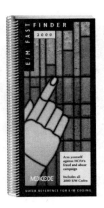

Quick and Easy Billing Audit Templates and Tips

2000 15-Minute Auditor
ISBN 1-56337-330-0

(Item #3104)   **$89⁹⁵**
Available September 1999

This portable, easy-to-use workbook provides templates and tips for front line health care professionals who want to make quick, random audits of coding and documentation operations to ensure their practice stays in compliance. You'll be able to spot activities that may result in fines or delayed reimbursement and initiate corrective action.

- **Quick audits.** Clear and easy-to-find instructions on how to do a "15-minute" audit.
- **Case Studies.** Illustrates common and unusual circumstances to help perform audits more quickly and with confidence.
- **Solutions.** Recommended solutions to specific compliance problems.
- **List of Frequently Asked Questions.** Gives you a head start on the auditing process.
- **Glossary of Auditing Terms.** Clarifies the subject and processes.
- **Convenient and Portable.** 6"x9" format makes it easy to take this book with you wherever you go.

Ensure the E/M Codes You are Reporting are Correct

2000 E/M Fast Finder
ISBN 1-56337-335-1

(Item #2752)   **$29⁹⁵**
Available January 2000

With this portable, easy-to-use, reference you can be assured E/M codes are correct before reporting patient encounters. Quick reference graphs make selecting the correct level of service easy. And the convenient size means you can take it wherever you go to make compliance a part of your daily activity.

- **NEW!** **Updated with 2000 E/M codes.** So you are using the most current codes.
- **Organized by Site of Service (Office, Hospital, Emergency, etc.).** Quickly find the exact range of E/M codes you need.
- **Quick Reference Graphs.** Easily check the level of history, exam, and medical decision-making to find the right E/M code.
- **Convenient.** Pocket size and durable pages make it ideal for the examination room.

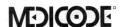

Medicode, 5225 Wiley Post Way, Suite 400, Salt Lake City, UT 84116 • 801.536.1000 • FAX 801.536.1011

ORDER TOLL FREE OR CALL FOR A FREE CATALOG 800.999.4600
AVAILABLE FROM YOUR MEDICAL BOOKSTORE OR DISTRIBUTOR.

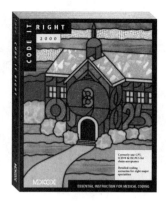

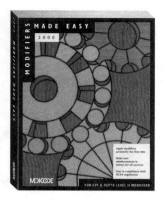

Help Your Office Master the Art of Coding!

2000 Code It Right
ISBN 1-56337-333-5

(Item #2750) $59⁹⁵
Available December 1999

Effective coding involves so much more than just looking up the correct codes or having all your documentation. It requires a thorough understanding of ICD-9, CPT, HCPCS, and DRG codes. *Code It Right* will give you that understanding of codes, coding rules and procedures, and coding techniques that maximize reimbursement and speed payment. No matter what your experience level, it is an excellent tool for the medical coder.

- **NEW! Overview of ICD-10-CM.** Helps you prepare for implementation.
- **NEW! Overview of outpatient surgery facility coding.** Broaden your coding knowledge to stay competitive.
- **Updated Annually with CPT, ICD-9-CM, HCPCS, and Medicare Changes.** Information is always up-to-date.
- **Actual Coding Scenarios with and without answers.** So you can test your skills.
- **Expert Advice.** Covers coding issues for CPT, ICD-9, and HCPCS, including E/M, Anesthesia, Surgery, Pathology, and more to help you code more accurately.
- **Includes examples of correctly completed HCFA-1500 forms.** So you can check for accuracy—before submitting.
- **Textbook Format.** Objectives are stated at the front of each section and discussion questions appear at the end. Makes a great teaching tool.

5 CEUs from AAPC

Apply Modifiers Easily and Accurately

2000 Modifiers Made Easy
ISBN 1-56337-346-7

(Item #4076) $79⁹⁵
Available December 1999

One of the top 10 billing errors is incorrect or missing modifiers. And billing errors mean rejected claims, which means you could be losing money. *Modifiers Made Easy* gives you everything you need to apply modifiers accurately, the first time.

Using modifiers correctly can maximize your reimbursement. And with HCFA looking into inappropriate use of modifiers in Medicare billing, it will help you stay in compliance as well.

- **NEW! Updated with 2000 Codes.** Provides clear definitions and coding tips for all CPT and HCPCS Level II modifiers—so you know you are applying the right code.
- **NEW! Updated real-life clinical examples with completed HCFA-1500 claim forms.** Helps you bill the correct modifier and reduce claims denials.
- **EXCLUSIVE! Common errors listed for each modifier.** Avoid mistakes which could result in delays, denials, or penalties.
- **EXCLUSIVE! Decision-Tree Flow Charts.** Helps you choose the correct modifier when more than one could apply.
- **CPT Modifiers Arranged by Type of Service:** E/M, Anesthesia, Surgery, etc. Quickly find the applicable modifier. Now includes cross-references between sections.
- **HCPCS Level II Modifiers Arranged Alphabetically.** Identify the right modifier at a glance.
- **Special hospital section lists outpatient-applicable modifiers.** Zero in on just the modifiers you need for outpatient services.

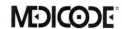

Medicode, 5225 Wiley Post Way, Suite 500, Salt Lake City, UT 84116 • 801.536.1000 • FAX 801.536.1011

ORDER TOLL FREE OR CALL FOR A FREE CATALOG 800.999.4600
AVAILABLE FROM YOUR MEDICAL BOOKSTORE OR DISTRIBUTOR.

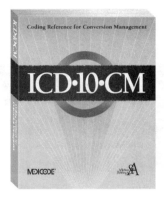

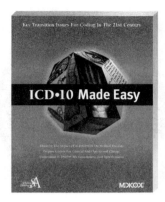

Evaluate how ICD-10-CM will Affect Your Practice

2000 ICD-10-CM
ISBN 1-56337-336-X

(Item #3012) **$79.95**

ICD-10-CM is the coding system that will replace *ICD-9-CM*. This unabridged code set allows you to familiarize yourself with all of the codes of your specialty, and begin formulating your plans for conversion to *ICD-10-CM*.

- **Detailed Introduction.** Explains how implementation will affect practices and how this book can be used as a management tool.
- **Official Guidelines.** Provides official government text in both the index and tabular sections.
- **ICD-10-CM Codes.** Complete *ICD-10-CM* tabular section and index.
- **Streamlined Format.** We guarantee you'll find our version of *ICD-10-CM* to be easy to use.
- **Availability.** Product will be available eight weeks after the government finalizes the *ICD-10-CM* code set (fourth quarter approval likely).
- **Prepare for the Future.** *ICD-10-CM* codes are **not** valid for current claim submission.

ICD-10 Primer Guides You Through Implementation Issues

ICD•10 Made Easy
ISBN 1-56337-237-1

(Item #2671) **$79.95**
Available Now

Learn the potential impact *ICD-10-CM* will have on your practice. This one-of-a kind narrative reference helps you understand the historical, medical, and statistical reasons why *ICD-10-CM* and *ICD-10-PCS* were developed.

- **Outline of Changes.** Examine each chapter of *ICD-9-CM* and discover how it will change under *ICD-10-CM*. Learn how the federal government's clinical modifications will affect you.
- **Documentation List.** Review our detailed list to learn what diagnoses will require more documentation under *ICD-10-CM* than they do under *ICD-9-CM*.
- **Implementation Issues.** Learn how to prepare information systems and other departments for the coming code changes.
- **Procedural Coding Systems.** Learn about the characteristics and complexities of CPT-5 and ICD-10-PCS.

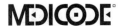

Medicode, 5225 Wiley Post Way, Suite 400, Salt Lake City, UT 84116 • 801.536.1000 • FAX 801.536.1011

ORDER TOLL FREE OR CALL FOR A FREE CATALOG 800.999.4600
AVAILABLE FROM YOUR MEDICAL BOOKSTORE OR DISTRIBUTOR.

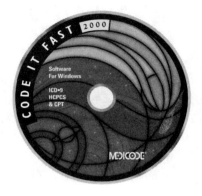

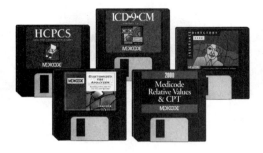

Get ICD-9, CPT and HCPCS Level II Codes—All on One Disk

1999-2000 ICD•9 Code It Fast
ISBN 1-56337-337-8
(Item #3230) **$99⁹⁵**

1999-2000 ICD•9, CPT & HCPCS Code It Fast
ISBN 1-56337-338-6
(Item #3220) **$199⁹⁵**

Windows 95™ or Windows NT 4.x, 8 MB RAM, 15 MB available hard disk space. 486 or Pentium recommended. For single user license only. Call for multi-user pricing.

Get all the features of the ICD-9, CPT, and HCPCS Level II code books in one convenient electronic format. Quickly look up codes in the index with fast search capabilities.

- **NEW! Available on CD-ROM.** The CD format allows for streamlined installation and more convenient storage.
- **Access codes electronically.** Look up ICD-9 codes in Volume 1 or 3, CPT codes, and HCPCS Level II codes.
- **Look Up Index Entries.** Enter key words and quickly view the matches in the ICD-9, CPT, or HCPCS index.
- **Color Coding Symbols.** Symbols for ICD-9, CPT, and HCPCS codes help you code quickly and easily.
- **Customize.** Sticky notes allow you to add your own comments to any code.
- **Annotations.** Explanations of diagnoses, supplies, and drugs help clarify code use.
- **Windows™ Compatible.** Copy codes and descriptions and reference information to the Windows clipboard for use in other Windows™ applications.

ASCII Files—Reliable Data From a Trusted Source

ICD•9 Vols. 1&3
(Item #3900) **$249⁹⁵**
Available September 1999

CPT & RVUs
(Item #3902) **$279⁹⁵**
Available January 2000

HCPCS Level II
(Item #3906) **$349⁹⁵**
Available January 2000

Insurance Directory
(Item #2850) **$229⁹⁵**
Available October 1999

Customized Fee Analyzer
Customized for your zip and specialty
Call for information.

With one of the industry's largest databases and patented methodologies, Medicode provides you with the best data. Our data files save you time and increase accuracy. No more updating your database a code at a time, just load the data file into a spreadsheet, database, or other application capable of reading text files.

- **NEW! 2000 Codes.** Each file is updated with the most current data.
- **Data Only Delivery.** Allows you to flow data into other applications and manipulate the data.
- **Value-Added Information.** ASCII files contain proprietary and clinically enhanced data.
- **Multiple-user Pricing.** Call for multi-user pricing.

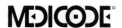

Medicode, 5225 Wiley Post Way, Suite 500, Salt Lake City, UT 84116 • 801.536.1000 • FAX 801.536.1011

ORDER TOLL FREE OR CALL FOR A FREE CATALOG 800.999.4600
AVAILABLE FROM YOUR MEDICAL BOOKSTORE OR DISTRIBUTOR.

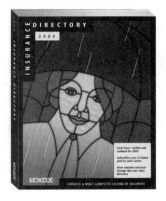

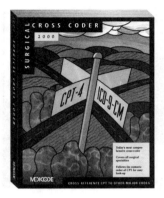

Add 5,000 Insurance Companies to Your Files Instantly

2000 Insurance Directory
ISBN 1-56337-329-7

(Item #2756) $59⁹⁵
Available October 1999

ASCII File*
ISBN 1-56337-284-3

(Item #2850) $349⁹⁵
Available October 1999

Get your claims in the right hands the first time. The majority of insurance companies experienced some change this past year in address, phone and fax numbers. For timely and accurate payment of claims, having a current edition of *Insurance Directory* is essential.

Medicode's exclusive features make our directory the market's largest and its #1 choice (ranking verified by market wholesalers).

- **NEW! Updated.** More than 5,000 updated insurance company listings.
- **More State-Specific Listings.** We list payers, national and local, both alphabetically and by state.
- **Know Which Payers Use HCPCS Codes.** We tell you which payers process HCPCS Level II codes on claims. No more guessing.
- **Electronic Claims Submission.** More than 1,100 carriers now accept claims electronically. We tell you which ones.
- **Most Accurate.** All entries have been contacted and verified for 2000.

Today's Most Comprehensive Cross Coder

2000 Surgical Cross Coder
ISBN 1-56337-326-2

(Item #2747) $139⁹⁵
Available December 1999

You face a constellation of codes and coding systems. How do you connect? This comprehensive and illustrated coding tool links more than 4,000 CPT surgical codes to their corresponding diagnostic, procedure and supply codes. Based on sound clinical assumptions and with the input of extensive data and clinical expertise, the *Surgical Cross Coder* provides a one-source cross coding book to simplify medical coding.

- **Organized by CPT Code.** CPT codes are listed numerically for quick reference.
- **Official Code Descriptions.** Lets you code accurately by providing detailed information.
- **Detailed Illustrations.** Visually orient yourself to the activity being described.
- **Notations.** Reminds you to seek out the causes of infection, their manifestations, and underlying diseases.
- **Variety of Code Sets.** Applicable ICD-9-CM, HCPCS, and ADA codes are included to save you from having to have a number of books open at your desk at one time.
- **Softbound.** Durable book without the weight and expense of a hardbound text.

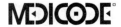

Medicode, 5225 Wiley Post Way, Suite 500, Salt Lake City, UT 84116 • 801.536.1000 • FAX 801.536.1011

ORDER TOLL FREE OR CALL FOR A FREE CATALOG 800.999.4600
AVAILABLE FROM YOUR MEDICAL BOOKSTORE OR DISTRIBUTOR.

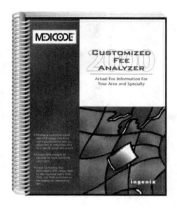

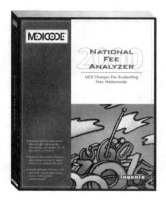

Determine Competitive and Accurate Fees

2000 Customized Fee Analyzer
Available December 1999

One Specialty		All CPT Codes ASCII	
(Item #2574)	$249.95	(Item #2591)	$599.95
Two Specialty		**One Specialty ASCII**	
(Item #2575)	$299.95	(Item #2583)	$459.95
All CPT Codes		**Two Specialty ASCII**	
(Item #2582)	$399.95	(Item #2589)	$529.95

A fair and defensible fee schedule based on your area's actual charge data is a tremendous advantage when determining fees and reimbursement. *Customized Fee Analyzer* takes charge information from your area and puts it into a customized report for your organization.

- **See your area's charges.** Provides you with your area's 50th, 75th, and 95th percentiles of charges, ensuring adequate data to determine accurate and defensible fees.
- **Relative values.** Provides you with trusted relative values to determine relative value based fees.
- **Negotiate your fee schedule.** Have area specific information to compare and contrast proposed fees and reimbursement.
- **Average indemnity allowable.** See the estimated amount being paid in your specific area.
- **Follow-up days.** See what commercial payers typically allow for follow-up days.
- **Trusted data.** Specific charge data is taken from regional-specific database containing more than 27 million covered lives.

Know What Physicians Across the Nation are Charging

2000 National Fee Analyzer
ISBN 1-56337-332-7

(Item #2503) $149.95
Available Febuary 2000

Having actual charge data to benchmark your fees is imperative in today's competitive health care market. *National Fee Analyzer* provides you with national averages of usual, customary, and reasonable (UCR) charge data. With data from more than 27 million covered lives, you can be assured of an accurate and comprehensive tool to help you determine competitive fees and reimbursement.

- **EXCLUSIVE! Database of more than 27 million covered lives.** Guarantees an accurate picture of fees with the largest and most statistically valid fee database.
- **Adjust data for your area.** *National Fee Analyzer* gives you conversion factors to estimate your specific area's fees.
- **National fee ranges.** Gives average national fee information for the 50th and 75th percentiles of charges.
- **Fee information for all CPT codes.** Provides fee information for all current CPT codes, based on national averages.
- **Know what codes you are valuing.** *National Fee Analyzer* is equipped with full CPT descriptions so you have a one-source reference for determining fees and reimbursement.
- **Relative values.** Determine fees based on the time and skill it takes to perform a procedure.
- **Determine Medicare reimbursement.** We give you the Medicare reimbursement rates with geographical adjustment factors so you can assure correct Medicare reimbursement.

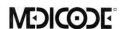

Medicode, 5225 Wiley Post Way, Suite 500, Salt Lake City, UT 84116 • 801.536.1000 • FAX 801.536.1011

Quick Guide to Physician Fraud & Abuse Prevention

MEDICODE®

Copyright © 2000 Ingenix Publishing

First Printing May 2000

First Edition — May 2000

All rights reserved. Printed in the United States of America. No part of this publication may be reproduced or transmitted in any form or by any means, electronic or mechanical, including photocopy, recording, or storage in a database or retrieval system, without the prior written permission of the publisher.

ISBN 1-56337-371-8

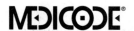

5225 Wiley Post Way, Suite 500
Salt Lake City, UT 84116-2889

Publishing Staff

Publisher	*Susan P. Seare*
Associate Medical Director	*Thomas G. Darr, MD, FACEP*
Senior Director of Publishing	*Lynn Speirs*
Product Manager	*André Hicks*
Project Editor	*Kimberli Turner*
Clinical Editor	*Bonnie G. Schreck, CCS, CCS-P, CPC, CPC-H*
Desktop Publishing Specialist	*Kerrie Hornsby*
Editorial Assistant	*Lisa Singley*

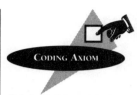

This book does not replace the CPT, ICD•9•CM, HCPCS Level II, or other coding system books.

Medicode Notice
This publication is designed to be an accurate and authoritative source regarding fraud and abuse prevention. Every effort has been made to verify accuracy and the information is believed reliable at the time of publication. This publication is made available with the understanding that the publisher in not engaged in rendering legal or other services requiring a professional license. Offices that have been contacted or notified by public or private payers about suspected fraudulent or abusive practices should seek appropriate professional legal counsel.

Contents

Introduction 1
   Fraud and Abuse Overview 2
   Time Line for Fraud and Abuse Legislation 4
   Fraud and Abuse Control Program 8
   Penalties for Fraud and Abuse 10
   Administrative Remedies 10
   Exclusions 10
   Civil Monetary Penalties 11
   Criminal Penalties 12
   Beneficiary Incentive Program .12
   Anti-Kickback Statute 12
   Price Reductions 13
   Hospital Incentives 14
   Self-Referral Prohibition 15
   Fraud Control: Medicare's Initiatives for Enforcement 16
   Fraud Alerts 17
   Special Advisory Bulletins 18
   Operation Restore Trust (ORT) .18
   Medicare Integrity Program 19
   Medicare Compliance Plans 20
   Establishment of an Internal Compliance Program 21
   Conclusion 27

Administrative Issues 29
   Advanced Beneficiary Notification 29
   Billing Company's Compliance Plan 30
   Compliance Officer 30
   Compliance Plan Development .31
   Contracts With A Billing Company 32
   Cost and Risk HMOs 32
   Financial Relationship Defined .33
   Going Solo and Participation 33

Medicare Participation and Group Practices 34
Medicare Secondary Payer (MSP) and Employer Size 34
New Ownership, Old Participation Agreement 34
"Opt Out" Affidavits 35
Opting Out of Medicare 36
Private Contract 36
Professional Associations and Participation Agreements . . .36
Rental Space in Physicians Offices 37

Audits & Monitoring 41
Audit Investigation 41
Audit Reports 41
Audit Resources 43
Audit Sample Size 44
Audit Sources 44
Auditing an In-Office Laboratory 45
E/M Documentation Requirements 45
Employee Performing Audit Functions 48
Initial Audit 48
Legal Audit 50
Monitoring Risk Areas 50
Monitoring Tools 51
Recommended Frequency of Self-Audits 52

Billing Policies 53
Balance Billing 53
Billing for Phone Calls 54
Billing Referral Services 55
Care Plan Oversight and Group Practices 56
Care Plan Oversight/Hospice 56
Care Plan Oversight Signatures .56
CCI Updates 57
Claim Form Signatures 57
Clinical Psychologist and Clinical Social Workers and E/M
    Codes 57
Conscious Sedation 58
Covered Visit with Preventive Care 59
Diagnostic Coding and the Nonphysician Practitioner 61
Different Payer, Different Charge? 61
HCFA-1500 Submission Requirements 62

Hospital Observation During Global Surgical Period 63
If Item 20 Is Blank 63
Incident To/Leased Nonphysicians 63
Injections 67
In-Office Oral Medications 67
In-Office Supplies 68
Item 9 and Nonparticipating Providers 70
Leaving Blanks on the HCFA-1500 Claim Form 70
Limited Licensed Practitioners 71
Linking Requirement 71
Misleading Suppliers' Advice 72
Nursing Facility Admissions and Other Outpatient
    Service Codes 73
Office Visits for Pneumococcal Pneumonia Vaccine
    (PPV) 73
Plan of Care on File 73
Postoperative Care/Second Physician 73
Prolonged Services 75
Signature Required 76
Stand-By Services 76
Written Billing Policies 76

Coding Policies **79**
Assumption Coding 79
Bundling Lesion Excision and Repair Codes 79
CCI's Effect on Claims 80
Consultations vs. Visits 81
CPO Requirement 81
CPO/Two Physicians 82
Critical Care 82
Cystourethroscopy and Ureteral Catheterization 83
Dictation and Time 83
E/M Based on Time 84
E/M: New vs. Established Patient 85
From Observation to Inpatient Status 85
Hospital Admissions 85
Immunizations 86
Incomplete Colonoscopy 86
Interpretation of Purified Protein Derivative of
    Tuberculin (PPD) 86

Modifier -80 86
"Mutually Exclusive" Policy 87
Observation Unit Visits 87
Previous History and Physical 88
Same-Day E/M Services 88
Sentinel Node Biopsy 89
Two Admission Visits 90
Two Visits, Same Day 90
"Unbundling" Defined 90
Using ED History 91

Coverage Issues **93**
Carrier Bulletins 93
Chiropractic Coverage 93
Covered Visit with Preventive Care 93
Diabetes Coverage 95
Dietitians' Services 96
Locum Tenens 96
Medical Necessity Denials 99
Noncovered Services and Supplies 101
Nonphysician Practitioners 103
Optometrist Services 103
Outside Lab Orders 104
Pap Smears 105
Physician Orders and Pneumococcal Pneumonia
    Vaccine (PPV) 105
Physician Referral 106
Pneumococcal Pneumonia Vaccine (PPV) and the Limiting
    Charge 106
Podiatry in Nursing Homes 107
PPV and Part A 107
RNs and PPV 107
Second Opinions 108
Telephone Orders 108
Telephone Referrals 108
Treating Relatives 108
Vaccination Status for Pneumococcal Pneumonia
    Vaccine (PPV) 110

Legislaton/Legal Issues 111

A Definition of "Overpayment" .111
Anti-Kickback Statute and Referral Prohibitions 112
Attorney-Client Privilege 113
Attorney's Role in Compliance 113
Beneficiaries and Fraud and Abuse 114
Civil Investigative Demand 115
Civil Monetary Penalties 116
Collections and the Limiting Charge 120
Consultants' Advice 120
Diagnostic Tests and Medical Necessity 120
Exclusion from Federal Health Care Programs 122
False Claims 124
Fraud and Abuse Differentiated .125
Fraud and Abuse Organizations .125
Fraud by a Billing Company 126
Healthcare Integrity and Protection Data Bank 127
Hospital Referrals and the Law .128
Improper Physician Certifications of Medical Necessity . .129
Inappropriate Certifications of Medical Necessity 129
Investment Interests 130
Laundering of Monetary Instruments 131
Limiting Charge Compliance Program 131
Medical Necessity Liability 132
Most Favored Nation Clauses 132
Observation Care 132
Professional Courtesy Discounts 133
Qui Tam 133
Reacting to a Search Warrant 134
Record Retention 135
Sanctions 135
"Standing Order" Defined 136
Waiving the Deductible and Copayment 136
When an Employee Commits Fraud 137

Payment Policies 139

Admission for Observation 139
Billing Anesthesia 139
Charge limits 140
Colorectal Screening 140

Diagnostic Tests 141
EGHP and Secondary Payer Rules 141
Fee Schedule Data Base 141
"Free" Pneumococcal Pneumonia Vaccine
    (PPV) Shots 142
"Incident To" Defined 142
Modifier -22 and Payment 143
Multiple Endoscopies 143
No Set Fee 145
Pneumococcal Pneumonia Vaccine 145
Psychotherapy and E/M Codes .146

Index **147**

Introduction

Medicode's *Quick Guide to Physician Fraud and Abuse Prevention* is a unique reference tool providing answers to physicians' most commonly asked fraud and abuse and compliance questions. It addresses questions ranging from coding, billing, and administrative issues to audits, self-monitoring, and legislation and legal issues affecting physician practices.

This product grew out of physicians' increasing interest in fraud and abuse issues, which has been spurred in recent years by the federal government's intensified efforts to detect, control, and prosecute health care provider's violations against the federal government. As fraud and abuse continues to consume an estimated $20 to $30 billion in Medicare funds each year, the government's determination to crack down on offenders has increased.

The government has taken action on both legislative and enforcement fronts. The Health Insurance Portability and Accountability Act of 1996 made all health care fraud a federal offense and authorized federal law enforcement agencies to find and prosecute violators. Both the Health Care Financing Administration (HCFA) and the Office of the Inspector General (OIG) began issuing fraud alerts, and began generating programs such as the Department of Health and Human Service's (HHS) Operation Restore Trust, which focuses on areas at high risk for fraud.

On the judicial front, a shift from criminal to civil penalties occurred for cases involving health care fraud and abuse. The stiffer monetary penalties available in civil cases and a less cumbersome burden of proof were two of the incentives driving this trend. Others came in the form of laws that allowed those reporting fraud and/or abuse to receive a financial incentive to

FACT

Fraud and abuse continues to consume an estimated $20 to $30 billion in Medicare funds each year.

Quick Guide to Physician Fraud and Abuse Prevention

become "whistleblowers" on violators, intensifying the growth in civil suits against physicians.

As both government and media attention have become more sharply focused on Medicare fraud and abuse, physicians have become alarmed at their audit liability risk. Medicare continues to establish more complex coding, billing, and payment policies than ever before, and physicians are struggling to keep up policies and procedures that are constantly changing.

Fraud and Abuse Overview

Both fraud and abuse can result in Medicare payment to which there is no entitlement, but fraud and abuse differ in degree. Abuse is the lesser offense.

HCFA defines abuse as incidents or practices that are not consistent with sound medical, business, or fiscal practices, such as the provision of medically unnecessary care, or care that fails to meet professionally recognized standards of care. These activities may directly or indirectly result in inappropriate costs to the Medicare program. It is considered a case of abuse when Medicare makes payments for items or services for which there is no legal entitlement and the provider has not knowingly and intentionally misrepresented facts to obtain that payment. It cannot be proven that the abusive acts were committed knowingly, willingly, and intentionally.

The following questions can help determine whether a practice is considered to be abusive:

- Is the service/supply medically necessary?
- Is the service/supply appropriate according to professionally recognized standards?
- Has a fair price been charged for the service/supply?

If the answer to any of these questions is no, abuse has occurred.

Fraud is an intentional deception or misrepresentation made by an individual who knows that the false information reported

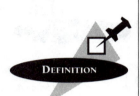

DEFINITION

Abuse
Incidents or practices that are not consistent with sound medical, business, or fiscal practices.

Fraud
An intentional deception or misrepresentation made by an individual who knows that the false information reported could result in an unauthorized benefit to himself/herself or another person.

Introduction

could result in an unauthorized benefit to himself/herself or another person.

Fraud takes many forms, including the following:

- Billing for services or supplies that were not provided
- Unbundling, i.e., coding individual components of a procedure separately when only a single code is necessary to describe the service provided (this may also be abuse if the individual performing coding duties is not educated or is unfamiliar with unbundling issues)
- Upcoding, i.e., misrepresenting the service provided, such as coding for an office consultation requiring a comprehensive history and examination and medical decision making of high complexity (CPT code 99245) when in reality, an office visit requiring a problem-focused history and examination and straightforward decision making was actually provided (CPT code 99201)
- Misrepresenting the diagnosis for the patient in order to justify the services or equipment provided
- Altering claims to obtain a higher payment amount
- Deliberately applying for duplicate payments (e.g., billing Medicare and the patient for the same service, or billing both Medicare and another payer to receive two payments)
- Prohibited completion of the certificate of medical necessity (CMN) form by suppliers
- Soliciting, offering, or receiving a kickback, bribe, or rebate
- Misrepresenting the services provided, the amounts charged, the identity of the person who received the service, the date of service, etc.
- Claims involving collusion between the provider and a patient or between a supplier and a provider, resulting in higher costs or charges to the Medicare program

Quick Guide to Physician Fraud and Abuse Prevention

- Excessive referrals (If a large number of patients are referred to a particular ancillary facility, payers may look into whether the provider has a financial interest in that facility)
- Overuse of health care services
- Billing for noncovered services
- Breaches of assignment agreements or charge limitation amounts
- Providing patients with inferior products
- Signing blank prescriptions or certificates of medical necessity

Time Line for Fraud and Abuse Legislation

1972   *Fraud and Abuse Amendments*
Allowed exclusion from the Medicare program for individuals who knowingly and willfully submitted false claims, provided care that was not medically necessary, or was "grossly inferior" or charged.

1974   *Anti-Kickback Statute*
Allowed for the imposition of criminal penalties of up to $25,000 and/or imprisonment for up to five years per offense, in addition to exclusion from the Medicare and Medicaid programs.

1977   *Anti-Fraud and Abuse Amendments*
Increased penalty provisions for providers to not more than $25,000 and/or imprisonment for up to five years for each offense, in addition to exclusion from the Medicare and Medicaid programs. For the same crime, a patient may face a fine of up to $10,000 and/or imprisonment of up to one year. In 1980, the elements of "knowingly and willfully" were added as the criteria of intent to the Anti-Kickback provision.

1981   *Civil Monetary Penalties*
Allowed for the imposition of civil monetary penalties and assessments on any individual who

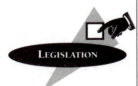

LEGISLATION

Anti-Kickback Statute
Allowed for the imposition of criminal penalties of up to $25,000 and/or imprisonment for up to five years per offense, in addition to exclusion from the Medicare and Medicaid programs.

Introduction

submitted a claim for services/supplies that were not provided as claimed, or for charges exceeding statutory standards. The scope of this legislation was broadened in 1987 to make employers accountable for staff billing errors.

1987　*Medicare and Medicaid Patient and Program Protection Act of 1987*
Allows the exclusion of health care providers, individuals, and businesses from receiving payment for services under Medicare, Medicaid, and other federal programs. Each sanction calls for assessments of up to double the violation amount, civil monetary penalties of up to $2,000 per violation, and exclusion from the Medicare program for up to five years.

1989–1996 *Self-Referral Prohibitions (Stark Law)*
Stark I provisions were included in the Omnibus Budget Reconciliation Act of 1989 (OBRA '89), which banned physicians from referring laboratory specimens to any entity with which the physician has a financial relationship. The effective date for Stark I was Jan. 1, 1992. Stark I was amended by OBRA '90 to exclude financial relationships between hospitals and physicians, unrelated to clinical laboratory services, and final regulations were issued in 1995. Stark I was expanded by OBRA '93 to include 10 other designated health care services. This expanded version is commonly referred to as "Stark II" and became effective Jan. 1, 1995.

1991–1993 *Safe Harbor Regulations*
These regulations, first implemented in 1991, specified 11 safe payment practices as exempt from the Anti-Kickback Statute. In 1992, the interim safe harbor rules were published, known as the Managed Care Safe Harbors. In 1993, seven additional safe harbors were proposed. In 1996, guidelines for safe harbor provisions to protect specific health care plans, such as HMOs and PPOs, were published. On

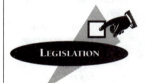

Safe Harbor Regulations
Eleven safe payment practices as exempt from the Anti-Kickback Statute.

Quick Guide to Physician Fraud and Abuse Prevention

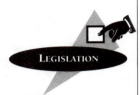

LEGISLATION

Health Insurance Portability and Accountability Act of 1996
- Establishes a Health Care Fraud and Abuse Control Account
- Imposes civil monetary penalties
- Imposes criminal penalties for "knowingly and willfully" defrauding any health care benefit program

1996

Nov. 19, 1999, published in the *Federal Register*, new safe harbor provisions were added, as well as clarification of the various aspects of the original safe harbor provisions.

Health Insurance Portability and Accountability Act of 1996 (HR 3103)
Combines the efforts of the Secretary of the Department of Health and Human Services (HHS) and the Attorney General in the establishment of a Fraud and Abuse Control Program. Establishes a Health Care Fraud and Abuse Control Account as an expenditure account within the Federal Hospital Insurance Trust Fund. Imposes civil monetary penalties for improper coding practices and for seeking reimbursement for services that are not medically necessary. Imposes criminal penalties for "knowingly and willfully" defrauding any health care benefit program. Congress declared war on all health care fraud and abuse and applied this provision to all payers. Health care fraud is now a "federal health care offense" with the full arsenal of federal law enforcement agencies available to find and punish violators. Fines are stiffer than in the past and transgressors face possible prison sentences. For purposes of this law, a health care benefit program is defined as "any public or private plan or contract, affecting commerce, under which any medical benefit, item, or service is provided to any individual and includes any individual or entity who is providing a medical benefit, item, or service for which payment is made under the plan or contract."

1997

Balanced Budget Act of 1997
The Balanced Budget Act (BBA) includes anti-fraud provisions that provide the government the ability to intervene in the battle against fraud, waste, and abuse. Some of these provisions are: Civil fines of up to $50,000 for each violation of the Anti-

Introduction

Kickback Statute, damages of up to three times the amount the illegal kickback paid, and monetary penalties for individuals who knowingly contract with sanctioned persons or entities. Two amendments of the BBA involve exclusions of sanctioned individuals from federally-funded programs for life if convicted of health-care related offenses three times. Family members may also be excluded to whom financial interests have been transferred by sanctioned individuals. The BBA also gives patients the right to request itemized Medicare bills from providers and the provider is required to honor their request in a specific amount of time.

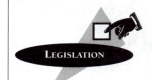

LEGISLATION

1998 *OIG's Provider Self-Disclosure Protocol*
In 1998, the OIG published the Provider Self-Disclosure Protocol, which states that providers have an obligation to institute a compliance plan to assist in detecting and preventing fraudulent, abusive, and wasteful activities. It also includes the need to implement procedures to inspect and resolve instances of non-compliance and the need for health care providers to investigate, assess, and identify potential losses suffered by federal health care programs and make full disclosures of non-compliance with these programs to the appropriate authorities. By self-disclosing instances of non-compliance, health care providers may be subjected to lower fines and penalties.

Provider Self-Disclosure Protocol
By self-disclosing instances of non-compliance, health care providers may be subjected to lower fines and penalties.

2000 *Compliance Program Guidance for Individual Physicians and Small Group Practices*
In 1999, in the *Federal Register*, solicitation was taken of information and recommendations, for the development of a compliance guidance program for individual physicians and small group practices. The OIG then determined by the information gathered that a compliance program should be developed for these entities that should follow along the lines of the Third Party Payer Compliance

Quick Guide to Physician Fraud and Abuse Prevention

Program Guidance. Also that it should contain the seven basic elements that are included in all of the other Compliance Guidances developed by the OIG. This Guidance should be released in 2000.

Fraud and Abuse Control Program

The Fraud and Abuse Control Program was established by the federal government. HHS's Office of the Inspector General (OIG), the Federal Bureau of Investigation (FBI), and the Department of Justice (DOJ) all share the responsibility for the investigation and prosecution of fraudulent providers. The OIG investigates suspected fraud and/or abuse and performs audits and inspections of HCFA programs. In carrying out its responsibilities, the OIG may request information or support from HCFA and its contractors. The OIG has access to HCFA's files, records, and data, as well as those of HCFA's contractors, which assists in their investigations of fraud and the development of cases. This office also has the authority to take action against individual health care providers in the form of civil monetary penalties (CMPs) and program exclusion and to refer to the DOJ for criminal or civil action. The OIG concentrates its efforts in the following areas:

- Conducting investigations of specific providers suspected of fraud, waste, or abuse to determine whether criminal, civil, or administrative actions are warranted

- Conducting audits, special analyses, and reviews for purposes of discovering and documenting Medicare and Medicaid policy and procedural weaknesses contributing to fraud, waste, or abuse, and making recommendations for corrections

- Conducting reviews and special projects to determine the level of effort and performance in health provider fraud and abuse control

- Participating in a program of external communications to inform the health care community, Congress, other organizations, and the public of the OIG's concerns and activities related to health care financing integrity

KEY POINT

The OIG concentrates its efforts in the following areas:

- Conducting investigations

- Conducting audits, special analyses, and reviews

- Conducting reviews and special projects to determine performance in health provider fraud and abuse control

- External communications to inform the public of the OIG's concerns and activities related to health care financing integrity

- Collecting and analyzing Medicare contractor and State Medicaid agency-produced information

- Participating to share techniques and knowledge on preventing health care provider fraud and abuse

Introduction

- Collecting and analyzing Medicare contractor and State Medicaid agency-produced information on resources and results
- Participating with other governmental agencies and private health insurers in special programs to share techniques and knowledge on preventing health care provider fraud and abuse

The FBI can investigate not only federal but also private payer cases of fraud, but does not have the authority to impose sanctions on providers. Both of these agencies may also refer cases to the DOJ, which can prosecute fraudulent providers for violations of federal criminal laws.

In addition, the program mandates the establishment of a national heath care fraud and abuse control program that coordinates the efforts of federal, state, and local law enforcement. These efforts include the following:

- Investigations, audits, evaluations, and inspections in the delivery of health care services and payment for those services
- Facilitation of the enforcement of statutes applicable to fraud and abuse in health care
- Providing education to providers by issuing fraud alerts, safe harbors, and advisory opinions
- Sharing information gathered from these efforts with public and private third-party payers

These efforts are not limited to Medicare and Medicaid but are applicable to any plan or program that provides health benefits.

To ensure continued funding of the anti-fraud efforts, a Health Care Fraud and Abuse Control Account was established. Created as an expenditure account within the Federal Hospital Insurance Fund, it is funded by the civil monetary penalties, fines, forfeitures, and damages assessed in health care cases, as well as by monetary gifts and bequests. These funds may also be used by the FBI for health care prosecution, audits, and provider and consumer education efforts.

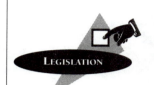

LEGISLATION

Health Care Fraud and Abuse Control Account
Funded by the civil monetary penalties, fines, forfeitures, and damages assessed in health care cases, as well as by monetary gifts and bequests. These funds may also be used by the FBI for health care prosecution, audits, and provider and consumer education efforts.

Penalties for Fraud and Abuse

Depending on the situation, abusive or questionable practices can be dealt with in a wide variety of ways ranging from educational contacts to conviction and jail time — and not just for Medicare violations. Under the provisions of the Fraud and Abuse Control Program, the application of certain criminal penalties for violations for fraud and abuse under Medicare and Medicaid were extended to similar violations in other federal health care programs. Federal health care programs are defined as "any plan or program that provides health benefits, which are funded directly, in whole or in part, by the United States' government."

Administrative Remedies

To correct abusive practices, administrative remedies may be initiated. These may include provider education, recovery of overpayments, withheld payments, or referrals to state licensing boards of medical and professional societies or to peer review organizations.

Exclusions

The Social Security Act allows for the permissive and mandatory exclusion of providers from participation in the Medicare and Medicaid programs as well as from receiving funds from Social Services and the Child Health Services Block Grants.

Mandatory exclusions require the termination of a provider or supplier for at least five years. They are initiated when a provider is convicted of criminal offenses related to the delivery of health care services, the abuse of a patient in relation to the delivery of a health care service or item, or controlled substances. Any individual who has been convicted on two or more previous occasions of health care related crimes will be permanently excluded.

Permissive exclusions are initiated by the OIG for criminal violations including, but not limited to, filing false claims for reimbursement, failure to grant HCFA or the OIG an immediate response for an inspection or investigation, and failure to

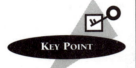

KEY POINT

Mandatory exclusions require the termination of a provider or supplier for at least five years.

provide information necessary to determine Medicare payment amounts. No payment for items or services will be provided to excluded providers. Application for reinstatement must be made to the OIG. Permissive exclusions may also be applied to any individual who has a direct or indirect ownership or controlling interest in a sanctioned entity and who knew or should have known about the activity serving as a basis for the conviction or exclusion. This provision is also applicable to an officer or manager of the entity who is in a position to have knowledge of potential fraudulent activity. Individuals who are at risk should be actively participating in all efforts to identify and correct errant billing practices and implement a compliance plan.

Civil Monetary Penalties

Civil monetary penalties may be imposed for false and fraudulent claims submitted to Medicare or any other federal health care program. These penalties have increased from a maximum of $2,000 for each item or service to $10,000 for each item or service. Additionally, the corresponding assessment has increased from twice to three times the amount claimed.

Any individual excluded from Medicare or a state health program who retains either direct or indirect ownership or control in an entity participating in Medicare, and any individual who knows or should have known the basis for an exclusion, or who is an officer or managing employee of the entity, is subject to a civil monetary penalty of not more than $10,000 for each day the relationship continues.

Civil monetary penalties of not more than three times the amount of the payments or $5,000, whichever is greater, will be imposed on physicians who falsely certify that a patient meets Medicare's requirements for home health care.

Additional practices that are subject to civil monetary penalties are improper coding and attempts to obtain reimbursement for services that are not medically necessary. Penalties of up to $10,000 may be imposed for each instance of medically unnecessary services.

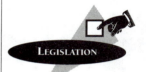

Civil Monetary Penalties may be imposed for false and fraudulent claims submitted to Medicare or any other federal health care program.

Quick Guide to Physician Fraud and Abuse Prevention

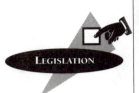

LEGISLATION

Criminal penalties of fines and up to 10 years in prison will be imposed for knowingly and willingly carrying out or attempting to carry out a scheme or artifice to defraud any health care benefit program or to obtain, by means of false or fraudulent pretense, money or property owned by or under the custody or control of any health care benefit program.

Criminal Penalties

Criminal penalties of fines and up to 10 years in prison will be imposed for knowingly and willingly carrying out or attempting to carry out a scheme or artifice to defraud any health care benefit program or to obtain, by means of false or fraudulent pretense, money or property owned by or under the custody or control of any health care benefit program. If a violation results in serious bodily harm to a patient, a prison sentence of up to 20 years may be imposed. If a patient dies as the result of a violation, the provider could be imprisoned for life.

In addition, any individual convicted of a federal health care offense may be ordered to forfeit all real or personal property derived either directly or indirectly from proceeds traceable to the commission of the offense.

Fines and/or imprisonment are imposed of up to five years for the following activities involving a health care benefit program when they are committed "knowingly and willfully":

- Falsifying, concealing, or covering up any trick, scheme, or device
- Making false, fictitious, or fraudulent statements or representations
- Making or using any false writing or document knowing it contains false or fraudulent statements

Beneficiary Incentive Program

Another important feature of of fraud and abuse legislation is the establishment of a beneficiary incentive program to encourage the reporting of information about individuals or entities that are engaged in fraud and abuse activities against the Medicare program. Monetary rewards are offered if the information leads to a collection of at least $100.

Anti-Kickback Statute

The Medicare and Medicaid Anti-Kickback Statute provides as follows:

Introduction

"Whoever knowingly and willfully solicits or receives any remuneration (including any kickback, hospital incentive, or bribe) directly or indirectly, overtly or covertly, in cash or in kind, in return for referring a patient to a person for the furnishing or arranging for the furnishing of any item or service for which payment may be made in whole or in part under Medicare, Medicaid, or a state health care program, or in return for purchasing, leasing, or ordering, or arranging for or recommending purchasing, leasing, or ordering any good, facility, service, or item for which payment may be made in whole or in part under Medicare, Medicaid, or a state health program shall be guilty of a felony and upon conviction thereof, shall be fined not more than $25,000 or imprisoned for not more than five years, or both."

This law is within the exclusive jurisdiction of the Department of Justice (DOJ). Because of the complexities of the Anti-Kickback Statute and safe harbor rules, legal counsel is recommended for all business dealings of this nature.

Price Reductions

Rebates, discounts, and other price reductions may be in violation of the Anti-Kickback Statute since they induce the purchase of items or services payable by Medicare or Medicaid. Some types of arrangements may be permissible if they fall within what is known in legal circles as a "safe harbor," such as certain discounting practices. For purposes of this safe harbor, a "discount" is defined as the reduction in the amount that a seller charges a buyer for a good or service based on an arms-length transaction. In addition, the discount must be applicable to the original item or service at the time it is purchased or provided. This means a discount cannot be applied to the purchase of a different good or service other than the good or service on which the discount was earned. "Rebate" is defined as a discount not given at the time of sale.

For a discount program to be protected for Part B billing, certain factors must exist. The discount must be made at the time of the sale of the good or service and must be accurately reported on the claim form. Credit or coupon discounts that are redeemable

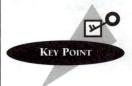

KEY POINT

Price Reductions
Rebates, discounts, and other price reductions may be in violation of the Anti-Kickback Statute.

Quick Guide to Physician Fraud and Abuse Prevention

directly from the seller may be protected if they are in compliance with the applicable standards in the safe discount harbor.

The following types of discounts are not protected:

- Rebates offered to beneficiaries
- Cash payments
- Items or services furnished free of charge or at a reduced rate in exchange for any agreement to buy a different item or service
- Price reductions applicable to one payer but not to Medicare or a state health care program
- Routine reductions or waivers of any coinsurance or deductible amount owed by a beneficiary

Hospital Incentives

Physician incentives, sometimes called "practice enhancements," are often used as tools to attract and retain physicians. The OIG has become aware that many of these programs are used to compensate physicians in return for referring patients to the hospital, a violation of the Anti-Kickback Statute. Some indicators of illegal activities include the following:

- Payment of any sort by a hospital each time a physician refers a patient to the hospital
- The use of free or significantly discounted office space or equipment (usually in facilities located near the hospital)
- Provision of free or significantly discounted billing, nursing, or other staff services
- Free training for a physician's staff in areas such as management, laboratory techniques, and ICD-9-CM and CPT coding
- Guarantees that supplement the physician's income if it fails to reach a predetermined level

ALERT

"Practice enhancements," are often used as tools to attract and retain physicians.

- Low interest or interest-free loans, or loans that are "forgiven" if a physician refers patients to the hospital
- Payment of the cost of the physician's travel and expenses for conferences
- Payment for a physician's continuing education courses
- Coverage on the hospital's group health plan at an inappropriately low cost to the physician
- Payment for services, including hospital consultations, that require few, if any, substantive duties by the physician, or payment for services in excess of the fair market value of the services provided

Self-Referral Prohibition

First effective on Jan. 1, 1992, the self-referral prohibition originally pertained to referring patients to clinical laboratories in which the physician had a financial interest. As of Jan. 1, 1995, the law was made effective for referrals for other designated health services as well. This means physicians who have a financial relationship with an entity (or with whom a member of the physician's immediate family has a financial relationship) may not make referrals to that entity for any of the following items and services:

- Clinical laboratory services
- Physical therapy services
- Occupational therapy services
- Home health services
- Inpatient and outpatient hospital services
- Durable medical equipment and supplies
- Radiology services including MRIs, CT scans, and ultrasound
- Outpatient prescription drugs
- Parenteral and enteral nutrients, equipment, and supplies
- Radiation therapy and supplies

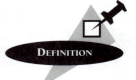

Self-referral Prohibition
Physicians who have a financial relationship with an entity may not make referrals to that entity.

- Prosthetics, orthotics, and prosthetic devices and supplies

A financial relationship can include ownership, interest investment, or a compensation arrangement. For services provided based on a prohibited referral, none of the entities listed above may bill Medicare, Medicaid, or the beneficiary for services. Violations are subject to civil monetary penalties of up to $15,000 for each service or exclusion from Medicare and Medicaid. For participation in cross-referral arrangements designed to sidestep the law, participants may be subject to civil monetary penalties of up to $100,000 per scheme.

Exceptions to the self-referral prohibition include the following:

- Physician referral to a member of the same legitimate group practice
- Services provided by organizations with prepaid plans and ownership in certain securities and mutual funds that are traded publicly
- Certain office ancillary services provided by solo practitioners and group practices

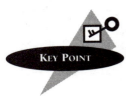

KEY POINT

A financial relationship can include ownership, interest investment, or a compensation arrangement.

Fraud Control: Medicare's Initiatives for Enforcement

Efforts to detect and eliminate fraud and abuse in the Medicare program have resulted in a great number and variety of initiatives to reach that goal. Some of these innovations include the establishment of fraud units at the carriers and durable medical equipment regional carriers (DMERCs); focused medical reviews; establishment of the National Provider System, which will assign a unique national provider identifier (NPI) to each provider; development of the Medicare Transaction System (MTS); and the Correct Coding Initiative, which incorporated a system of edits to detect unbundling. These efforts have also resulted in increased communication with providers and educational innovations, such as fraud alerts. In the future, expect to see innovations such as sophisticated anti-fraud computer technology.

Introduction

Fraud Alerts

Both HCFA and the OIG issue special fraud alerts to inform providers, payers, and the public of activities that are considered to be suspicious as fraudulent practices. These alerts also serve to warn providers and suppliers of the practices currently being investigated so they can examine their practices for any possible oversights and correct them.

Fraud alerts may be issued as National Fraud Alerts. The following Special Alerts have been issued since 1988. They address:

- Joint venture arrangements
- Routine waiver of Medicare Part B deductibles and copayments
- Prescription drug marketing practices
- Hospital incentives to referring physicians
- Arrangements for the provision of clinical laboratory services
- Home health fraud
- Medical services to nursing homes
- Provision of services in nursing facilities
- Fraud and abuse in nursing home arrangement with hospices
- Physician liability for certifications in the provision of medical equipment and supplies and home health services
- Rental or space in physician offices by persons or entities to which physicians refer

Special fraud alerts may also contain information regarding current fraudulent or abusive national trends that may be or are perceived to have the potential to become widespread. These fraud alerts identify only a particular activity or scheme that serves as a lead for fraud detection. They do not contain the names of individuals associated with that activity.

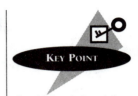

KEY POINT

Special fraud alerts inform providers, payers, and the public of activities that are considered to be suspicious as fraudulent practices.

Quick Guide to Physician Fraud and Abuse Prevention

Special Advisory Bulletins

Also issued by the OIG are Special Advisory Bulletins. Included in the Special Advisory Bulletins are the:

- Patient Anti-Dumping Statute
- The Effect of Exclusion From Participation in Federal Health Care Programs
- Gainsharing Arrangements and CMPs for Hospital Payments to Physicians to Reduce or Limit Services to Beneficiaries

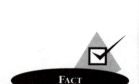

FACT

Operation Restore Trust (ORT)
Program savings from the first two years totaled $187.5 million in restitution, fines, settlements, and other identified overpayments.

Operation Restore Trust (ORT)

ORT is an anti-fraud program with several new anti-fraud and abuse approaches developed in 1995 by the Clinton administration. This program was a two-year demonstration in partnering with law enforcement agencies to target Medicare and Medicaid fraud in five of the largest states: California, Florida, New York, Texas, and Illinois. This consisted of more than a third of the nation's Medicare and Medicaid beneficiaries and led to record levels of criminal convictions, fines, exclusions, and a new collaborative way of approaching program integrity. Program savings from the first two years totaled $187.5 million in restitution, fines, settlements, and other identified overpayments.

An expansion of ORT was launched in 1997, which included:

- The use of sophisticated statistical methods to identify providers for investigations and audits
- The use of interdisciplinary teams to review individual facilities with unusually high Medicare reimbursement rates. Reviewers look both for facility-specific evidence and for indications of systemic problems
- Increased emphasis on concerted planning and conducting of investigations with the Department of Justice and other law enforcement agencies

Introduction

- Training and empowering state and local aging organizations and ombudsmen to detect and report fraud in nursing homes and in other settings
- Use of state survey officials who regularly monitor care in home health agencies and nursing homes to help identify inappropriate and fraudulent billing

ORT is a joint effort within the Department of Health and Human Services, involving the Office of the Inspector General, the Health Care Financing Administration, and the Administration on Aging.

Medicare Integrity Program

The Medicare Integrity Program (MIP) strengthens the ability of the Secretary of HHS to deter fraud and abuse. It allows for contracts with eligible private companies to perform the following functions:

- Review the activities of providers of items and services under the Medicare program, including medical, utilization, and fraud review
- Determine the appropriateness of payment under Part B
- Cost report auditing
- Develop and update lists of durable medical equipment that require prior authorization
- Educate providers, beneficiaries, and others regarding program integrity and quality assurance issues.

In addition, rather than being able to contract only with existing fiscal intermediaries (FIs) and carriers, MIP allows for the use of competition to obtain contract services for the best value.

At the present time, MIP functions are performed as part of claims processing by the FIs and carriers. Once MIP is implemented, they would no longer perform those functions unless they enter into a contract to do so.

Fact

MIP allows for the use of competition to obtain contract services for the best value.

Quick Guide to Physician Fraud and Abuse Prevention

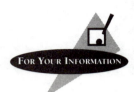

For Your Information

The Office of the Inspector General in the Department of Health and Human Services has developed compliance guidances for the following health care entities:

- Hospices
- Durable Medical Equipment, Prosthetics, Orthotics, and other suppliers
- Third-Party Medical Billing Companies
- Home Health Agencies
- Clinical Laboratories
- Hospitals
- Nursing Facilities

Medicare Compliance Plans

Providers who are found to be out of compliance with fraud and abuse laws involving billing and coding are often required to establish billing compliance programs to remedy their erroneous billing practices. In general, physicians can take proactive measures to improve the accuracy of their billing, including reviewing billing procedures, correcting any systemic weaknesses that could lead to erroneous or false claims, and establishing effective controls, such as a billing compliance program, to prevent future trouble.

The Office of the Inspector General in the Department of Health and Human Services has developed compliance guidances for the following health care entities:

- Hospices
- Durable Medical Equipment, Prosthetics, Orthotics, and other suppliers
- Third-Party Medical Billing Companies
- Home Health Agencies
- Clinical Laboratories
- Hospitals
- Nursing Facilities

In September of 1999, a notice was posted in the *Federal Register* for solicitation of information and recommendations for developing the physician program guidance. It is anticipated that the Compliance Program Guidance of Individual Practices and Small Group Practices will soon be announced by the OIG. Compliance programs ensure that physicians and billing staff know about and comply with Medicare rules and regulations and complete periodic reviews of compliance with the regulations. An effective compliance program can reduce the risk of civil and criminal action and reduce penalties if there is a problem, as well as help physicians avoid the negative press and business consequences of a fraud investigation. An additional benefit is that a strong system of internal controls, incorporating a sound compliance program, allows physicians to position their practices to be more successful.

Introduction

A compliance program needs to be integrated into daily operational procedures rather than exist as a paper document sitting on a shelf. Integrated controls produce benefits including operational efficiency and effectiveness, reliable management information, and compliance.

Compliance controls are needed to deal preemptively with all potential risks. A very basic step is to know what goes on in your organization. A legal and risk evaluation by other experts is a first step in helping to understand the current risks. Also, be aware of utilization statistics and know what are considered normal billing and utilization patterns based on diagnoses and procedure codes.

A compliance plan may also be considered a safety net in the event of a federal audit. It is a pattern of documentation or an audit trail that indicates an effort to comply with federal regulations in billing and coding practices for services rendered to a Medicare/Medicaid patient.

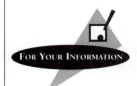

A compliance plan may be considered a safety net in the event of a federal audit.

Establishment of an Internal Compliance Program

Out of the Federal Sentencing Guidelines flow seven elements of what federal authorities deem an effective compliance program. These elements were developed for criminal prosecutions and are used in conjunction with a complex system of points. These common concepts will help to mitigate many adverse consequences in the event of a problem.

1. Development and distribution of written standards of conduct, as well as written policies and procedures that promote the health care organization's commitment to compliance (e.g., by including adherence to compliance as an element in evaluating managers and employees.

2. Designation of a chief compliance officer and other appropriate bodies (e.g., a corporate compliance committee) charged with the responsibility of operating and monitoring the compliance program.

3. Development and implementation of education and training programs for all affected employees.

4. Maintenance of a process, such as a hotline, to receive complaints, and the adoption of procedures to protect the anonymity of complainants and to protect whistleblowers from retaliation.

5. Development of a system to respond to allegations of improper/illegal activities and the enforcement of appropriate disciplinary action against employees who have violated internal compliance policies, applicable statutes, regulations, or requirements of federal, state, or private health plans.

6. The use of audits and/or other evaluation techniques to monitor compliance and assist in the reduction of identified problem areas.

7. Investigation and remediation of identified systemic problems and the development of policies addressing the non-employment or retention of sanctioned individuals.

Written Policies and Procedures:

Written policies and procedures should include areas that are specific to the physician's practice. These are:

- Standards of conduct
- Risk areas—risk assessment
- Medical necessity—reasonable and medically necessary services
- Anti-kickback and self-referral issues
- Claim development and submissions process
- Credit balances—bad debts
- Description of the coding check and balance process
- Payment processing (i.e., receipting, balancing, and documenting, etc.)
- Integrity of data systems
- Retention of records

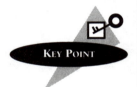

KEY POINT

Written policies and procedures should include areas that are specific to the physician's practice.

- Employee performance in relation to the compliance plan

Distribute billing and reimbursement policies annually among finance, admitting, and registration staff, billing personnel, physicians, coders, and others involved with the billing process. All employees would require a copy of standards of conduct and employee performance in relation to the compliance plan.

Compliance Officer/Committee:

Assign an individual within your organization or outsource the responsibility as compliance officer to oversee the compliance program. Whether you designate an individual with the sole responsibility of compliance officer, with responsibilities in addition to compliance officer, or whether you outsource the position will depend on the size of your organization. This person should be able to accept the responsibilities of:

- Overseeing and monitoring the compliance program
- Identifying components of the compliance plan and the individuals/departments involved in the implementation process
- Coordinating compliance efforts with individuals and departments to ensure that the elements of the compliance plan are carried out appropriately
- Reporting to the organization's governing body, CEO, and/or compliance committee
- Establishing methods to improve efficiency and quality of services and to reduce vulnerability to fraud, abuse, and waste
- Monitoring changes in laws and regulations
- Revising the compliance plan to adjust to the changing needs of the organization
- Reviewing employee's records to verify they understand the standards of conduct

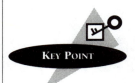

KEY POINT

Assign an individual within your organization or outsource the responsibility as compliance officer to oversee the compliance program.

Quick Guide to Physician Fraud and Abuse Prevention

- Developing and coordinating compliance-related education and training programs
- Developing and distributing compliance policies and procedures to all affected employees
- Ensuring that all relevant employees and management are knowledgeable of and comply with pertinent federal and state standards
- Ensuring that all employees involved in documentation, coding, billing, and reimbursement processes are well-informed of and comply with pertinent federal and state policies and procedures, as well as private payer requirements
- Communicating changes to the appropriate individuals/departments
- Ensuring that independent contractors and agents are aware of and abide by the requirements of the organization's compliance program
- Coordinating personnel issues to ensure that all employees, medical staff, and contracted individuals are not sanctioned
- Coordinating and assisting departments and/or department heads with any internal compliance audits and/or monitoring activities
- Investigating and acting on matters related to compliance, including internal investigations
- Overseeing any corrective actions
- Developing policies and procedures that encourage employees to report any fraud, waste, and/or abuse or compliance concerns without fear or reprisal

Education and Training:

The elements of the organization's compliance program should be emphasized. All personnel should receive pertinent training about federal and state statutes, regulations and guidelines, policies of private payers, and ethics. Other training may be more specific, such as detailing fraud and abuse laws, coding rules and guidelines,

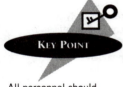

KEY POINT

All personnel should receive pertinent training about federal and state statutes, regulations and guidelines, policies of private payers, and ethics.

claim development and submission processes, and marketing practices that reflect current program standards. Any individual directly involved with any of these elements should be trained, including physicians, independent contractors, and other staff members.

Training should include:

- New physician orientation to coding and billing rules
- New staff orientation to coding and billing rules
- Programs for physicians
- Periodic training of staff related to coding, payment, and reimbursement accuracy

Developing Effective Lines of Communications

Issues that should be addressed when developing effective lines of communication are the development of an environment that encourages communication, providing several methods by which to communicate compliance-related concerns, and responding to compliance concerns.

Some communication components that are required to be in written policies and procedures are:

- Mechanisms to encourage effective communication among employees, compliance officer/committee, and all others involved in the organization
- A process for reporting questions, concerns, complaints, or suspected violations to the compliance officer/committee (e.g., hotline, e-mail, written notes)
- An independent reporting path outside the normal chain of command
- A guarantee to any employee or individual reporting questions, concerns, complaints, or suspected violations that, whenever possible, confidentiality will be maintained
- Non-retaliation policy

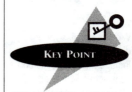

Effective Lines of Communication
The development of an environment that encourages communication, providing several methods by which to communicate compliance-related concerns, and responding to compliance concerns.

Quick Guide to Physician Fraud and Abuse Prevention

- A guarantee that questions, concerns, complaints, or suspected violations will be answered in a timely manner
- Suspected violations will be investigated
- A process for recording all compliance communications
- A method for evaluating the effectiveness of the established communications process

Enforcement of Standards through Well-Publicized Disciplinary Guidelines

Written policies for disciplinary action should include all employees and contractors of the physician organization. A course of action should take place when violators are identified. Any intentional or reckless disregard for policies and/or procedures of the compliance plan should subject individuals to disciplinary actions, which may include:

- Verbal warnings
- Written warnings
- Change in job title
- Suspension
- Privilege revocation
- Financial penalties
- Termination

The disciplinary action taken will depend on the violation committed. All employees should be subject to the same disciplinary action for similar offenses.

Auditing and Monitoring

Compliance plans need an initial audit to determine a baseline for developing the compliance plan. This will identify the risk areas associated specifically with the organization and determine how often areas should be audited and monitored.

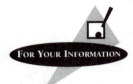

For Your Information

Written policies for disciplinary action should include all employees and contractors of the physician organization.

Compliance plans need an initial audit to determine a baseline for developing the compliance plan.

Introduction

The OIG has stated that an audit should be performed at least annually. Otherwise, audits could be performed quarterly, monthly, weekly, or as needed, depending on the risk areas identified by the initial audit and during the monitoring process.

Corrective Action

If misconduct is uncovered, steps should be taken, such as:

- Implementation of a corrective action plan
- Report to the appropriate governmental authority
- Referral to criminal and/or civil law enforcement authorities
- Notification of any discrepancies or overpayments

If any violation of criminal, civil, or administrative law is identified, the provider organization should be notified within 60 days. In order for the provider to qualify for less than double damages, according to the False Claims Act, the report must be provided to the government within 30 days. This will exhibit the provider's willingness to work with government authorities and may factor in determining administrative sanctions and financial penalties and damages.

Conclusion

Medicode's *Quick Guide to Physician Fraud and Abuse Prevention* is designed to give physicians and their office staff direction in resolving their fraud and abuse concerns. This book also provides you with the essential elements of a compliance plan that can assist in filling in any gaps that may exist in your current compliance or review processes. As you move through the course of evaluating and modifying your billing policies and procedures, and more compliance questions arise, this book will prove to be an invaluable reference tool.

The questions and answers in the *Quick Guide to Physician Fraud and Abuse Prevention* are divided into seven major subject

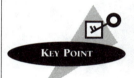

KEY POINT

In order for the provider to qualify for less than double damages, according to the False Claims Act, the report must be provided to the government within 30 days.

areas, and a detailed table of contents and an alphabetical index will help you quickly and easily locate the answers you need.

Note: These are the questions physicians and office managers ask most often concerning fraud and abuse. Be sure to browse through the entire book for an overview of issues you may need to consider in developing your own compliance plan or areas that may be trouble spots in your practice's billing procedures. Review the sections for an overview of the fraud and abuse programs, policies, legislation, and regulations affecting compliance today, as well as the recommended compliance plan elements from the federal sentencing guidelines.

Administrative Issues

Advanced Beneficiary Notification

What is the Advanced Beneficiary Notification (ABN) form of waiver of liability and when do I need to get it signed?

The "waiver of liability" provision, also known as the "limitation of liability," was established to protect the patient and the provider from unknowingly being liable for services that Medicare denies as medically unnecessary. The provision applies only to assigned claims for services that Medicare determines are not "reasonable or necessary." It does not apply to services or supplies that are denied because of Medicare exclusions (i.e., services never covered, such as bathroom safety equipment). The patient is responsible for payment of items and services not covered under the Medicare program.

Medicare determines liability based on who should have known that the services or supplies would be denied as medically unnecessary. If the patient was informed in advance that the services in question were not medically necessary, the patient would be held liable for the denied services. If the provider knew that Medicare generally denies a specific service as medically unnecessary, but the patient did not know, the provider is held liable for the service and may not bill the patient. If neither the provider nor the patient could have known that Medicare would deny the service as medically unnecessary, the Medicare program will pay if the service is otherwise covered.

Because coverage information and periodic advisories are sent out to providers, they are generally expected to know which services are likely to be denied. Therefore, unless an

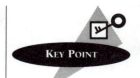

KEY POINT

Medicare determines liability based on who should have known that the services or supplies would be denied as medically unnecessary.

Quick Guide to Physician Fraud and Abuse Prevention

indication is received on the claim that the patient was informed that the service would likely be denied as medically unnecessary, Medicare will consider the provider liable for the denied service or supply.

If a provider renders a service or provides a supply that Medicare considers not medically necessary, the provider should notify the patient in writing before providing the service or supply that Medicare will deny the claim and that the patient will be responsible for the payment. Modifier -GA should be appended to the appropriate HCPCS code on the HCFA-1500 claim form when it is filed.

Billing Company's Compliance Plan

The billing company I use has indicated that they have a compliance plan. What information should I expect to receive from them regarding their compliance program?

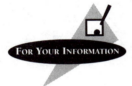

For Your Information

You should receive an outline of compliance plan issues that are directly related to your relationship with the billing company.

You should receive an outline of compliance plan issues that are directly related to your relationship with the billing company. Included in this outline should be items such as steps the billing company is taking to follow the rules and regulations of federally-funded programs and third-party payers, their policy on overpayments and underpayments, education and training on coding and reimbursement, and requirements of their employees who perform the coding and billing.

Compliance Officer

What skills and knowledge are required to perform the functions of compliance officer?

It is important to designate a compliance officer who has the authority to perform the duties required by the title. This individual should have self-confidence and be assertive enough to confront issues and influence behavior at all levels in a work place hierarchy. Personal character is important; he/she must have a high ethical standard. The

30

Administrative Issues

compliance officer also needs to possess strong written, verbal, and organizational skills, and be able to communicate to all individuals related to the compliance plan, such as legal counsel, executive management, and all employees in a highly functional manner. The individual should be familiar with all of the practice's functions, especially those related to billing and reimbursement. If misconduct or violations of the compliance plan are identified, he/she should have the ability to confront all individuals involved and take the necessary actions.

Compliance Plan Development

Since the federal government does not require physicians to implement a compliance program and has not yet developed compliance guidance for physicians, should our office go ahead and develop one anyway?

Yes. Although a Guidance will be available in the near future, a compliance plan will demonstrate to the government and third party payers that your practice is making every effort to be compliant with rules and regulations that prevent fraud, waste, and abuse in the health care industry. This may prevent your practice from receiving fines and penalties caused by overpayments and underpayments. The sooner the compliance plan is in place, the sooner your practice will be compliant.

What guidelines should we use?

The Guidelines from the OIG that most closely resemble how the compliance plan should work in a physician's office is the one developed for third-party billing companies. Although all of the Guidances contain the same seven elements that need to be included in a compliance plan, billing companies and physician offices perform their billing and reimbursement functions similarly, since they are both billing for physician practices.

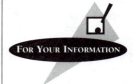

For Your Information

The sooner the compliance plan is in place, the sooner your practice will be compliant.

Contracts With A Billing Company

Is it important for a physician's office that contracts with a third party coding/billing company to understand the OIG Compliance Program Guidance for Third-Party Billing Companies?

Yes. This will enable the physician's office to understand if the coding/billing company is compliant with policies and is following a compliance program that will prevent fraud, waste, and abuse in federally-funded health care programs and with third-party payers. The physician's office may also prevent liability by recognizing any violations or misconduct that may be occurring unintentionally or knowingly by the billing company.

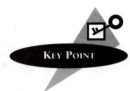

KEY POINT

The physician's office may also prevent liability by recognizing any violations or misconduct that may be occurring unintentionally or knowingly by the billing company.

Cost and Risk HMOs

Beneficiaries have difficulty distinguishing between cost and risk HMOs. What is the distinction between these two types of HMOs? How does this difference affect the beneficiary?

Beneficiaries enrolled in a risk HMO must receive all of their care through the plan's doctors, hospitals, and other health care providers, except for emergency care and unforeseen out-of-area care. This is referred to as being "locked in."

Beneficiaries enrolled in a cost HMO may choose to receive all of their care through the plan's doctors, hospitals, and other health care providers, or they may choose to receive their medical care from any other health care provider who participates in the Medicare program. However, if beneficiaries do not choose a health care provider in their plan, they are responsible for paying all of the coinsurance and deductibles associated with such out-of-plan care.

Administrative Issues

Financial Relationship Defined

What constitutes a financial relationship?

A physician has a financial relationship with an entity if he/she (or an immediate family member) has an ownership or investment interest in that entity or a compensation arrangement with the entity.

A physician's or family member's ownership/investment interest may be through equity, debt, or other means. It includes an interest a physician or family member has in an entity that does not itself provide designated health services, but which owns or holds an investment interest in an entity that does provide these services (e.g., an investment in a holding company).

A compensation arrangement exists when there is any arrangement in which payment of any kind passes between a physician (or immediate family member) and an entity. For example, a physician has a compensation arrangement with an entity if the entity pays the physician a salary or consulting fee. A compensation arrangement also exists if a physician pays an entity for items or services. These payments can be direct or indirect, overt or covert, in-cash or in-kind. The law does not regard as compensation a small list of specific payments, such as those meant to correct minor billing errors.

Because of the complexity of these contracts it is recommended that legal counsel review all of the practice's contractual agreements to assure compliance.

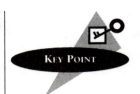

KEY POINT

A physician has a financial relationship with an entity if he/she (or an immediate family member) has an ownership or investment interest in that entity or a compensation arrangement with the entity.

Going Solo and Participation

I was practicing with a group that was participating, but recently decided to open an individual practice. Will I be considered participating or nonparticipating?

You may choose whether or not to participate at your individual practice without regard to the participation

33

Quick Guide to Physician Fraud and Abuse Prevention

status of the group. However, a contract must be filed for your individual practice if you choose to participate.

Medicare Participation and Group Practices

My partner and I are currently participating providers and we have decided to form a group. Will our group participation status automatically reflect participating?

No. A separate agreement must be filed on behalf of the group. The agreement binds all physicians with respect to any service billed by the group.

Medicare Secondary Payer (MSP) and Employer Size

Some MSP provisions are based on the size of the beneficiary's employer, but does Medicare consider the number of employees enrolled in the group health plan or the total number of employees when determining the size of the employer?

HCFA requires that the total number of employees (both full- and part-time) be considered in determining the application of the MSP provisions.

For the working aged provision, Medicare is secondary if the employer has 20 or more employees. For the disabled provision, Medicare is secondary if the employer has 100 or more employees. For the end-stage renal disease (ESRD) provision, the number of persons employed by the employer is irrelevant.

New Ownership, Old Participation Agreement

My professional association has changed ownership. As a result, we have been issued a new group provider number. Is it necessary to complete a new agreement?

Yes. If a participant receives a new provider number as a result of a change in ownership, it is necessary for the

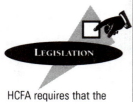

LEGISLATION

HCFA requires that the total number of employees be considered in determining the application of the MSP provisions.

Administrative Issues

participant to file a participation agreement on behalf of the newly assigned provider number.

"Opt Out" Affidavits

What is required in the Medicare "opt out" affidavit and where should it be filed?

To be valid, the affidavit must:

- Provide that the physician or practitioner will not submit any claim to Medicare for any item or service provided to any Medicare beneficiary during the two-year period beginning on the date the affidavit is signed

- Provide that the physician or practitioner will not receive any Medicare payment for any items or services provided to Medicare beneficiaries

- Be filed with all carriers who have jurisdiction over claims the physician or practitioner would otherwise file with Medicare and must be filed no later than 10 days after the first private contract to which the affidavit applies is entered into

- Be in writing and signed by the physician or practitioner

- Identify the physician or practitioner sufficiently that the carrier can ensure that no payment is made to the physician or practitioner during the opt out period. If the physician has already enrolled in Medicare, this would include the physician or practitioner's Medicare uniform provider number (UPIN) if one has been assigned. If the physician has not enrolled in Medicare, this must include the information necessary to be assigned a UPIN

Quick Guide to Physician Fraud and Abuse Prevention

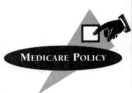

MEDICARE POLICY

Under the law, optometrists, chiropractors, podiatrists, dentists, or doctors of oral surgery are not permitted to opt out of Medicare.

Opting Out of Medicare

Who can "opt out" of Medicare under the provision in the Balanced Budget Act of 1997?

The physicians and practitioners permitted to "opt out" of Medicare under this provision include doctors of medicine and of osteopathy, physician assistants, nurse practitioners, clinical nurse specialists, certified registered nurse anesthetists, certified nurse midwives, clinical social workers, and clinical psychologists.

Under the law, optometrists, chiropractors, podiatrists, dentists, or doctors of oral surgery are not permitted to opt out of Medicare and provide services under private contract, nor are physical or occupational therapists in independent practice.

Private Contract

What is a "private contract" and what does it mean to a Medicare beneficiary who signs it?

As provided in the Balanced Budget Act of 1997, a "private contract" is a contract between a Medicare beneficiary and a physician or other practitioner who has "opted out" of the Medicare program for two years for all covered items and services he/she furnishes to Medicare beneficiaries. In a private contract, the Medicare beneficiary agrees to give up Medicare payment for services furnished by the physician or practitioner without regard to any limits that would otherwise apply to what the physician or practitioner could charge.

Professional Associations and Participation Agreements

My professional association has decided to join the Medicare Part B participation program. Is it necessary to complete an agreement for each group member?

No. Only one participation agreement is needed for the group.

Rental Space in Physician Offices

What arrangements are suspect when physicians rent office space to entities such as durable medical suppliers and mobile diagnostic suppliers?

The features of suspected rental agreements for space in the physician's offices that may be questionable are:

- The appropriateness of rental agreements
- The rental amounts
- Time and space considerations

Potentially areas that may violate the Anti-Kickback Statute and have indicators of unlawful activity include:

Appropriateness of Rental Agreements — The threshold inquiry when examining rental payments is whether payment for rent is appropriate at all. Payments of "rent" for space that has been traditionally provided for free or for a nominal charge as an accommodation between the parties for the benefit of the physicians' patients are suspect.

Rental Amounts — Rental amounts should be at fair market value, be fixed in advanced and not take into account, directly or indirectly, the volume or value of referrals or other business generated between the parties. Fair market value rental should not exceed the amount paid for comparable property. Moreover, where a physician rents space, the rate paid by the supplier should not exceed the rate paid by the physicians in the primary lease for

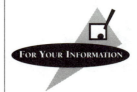

For Your Information

Rental amounts should be at fair market value, be fixed in advanced and not take into account, directly or indirectly, the volume or value of referrals or other business generated between the parties.

their office space, except in rare circumstances. Some examples of suspect arrangements include:

- Rental amounts paid in excess of amounts paid for comparable property rented in arms-length transactions between persons not in a position to refer business
- Rental amounts for subleases that exceed the rental amounts per square foot in the primary lease
- Rental amounts that are subject to modification more often than annually
- Rental arrangements that vary with the number of patients or referrals
- Rental amounts that are only paid if there are a certain number of federal health care program beneficiaries referred each month
- Rental amounts that are conditioned upon the supplier's receipt of payments from a federal health care program

Time and Space Considerations — Suppliers are only allowed to rent premises of a size and for a time that is reasonable and necessary for a commercially reasonable business purpose of the supplier. Rental of space that is in excess of a supplier's need makes suspect that the payments may be an indicator that the supplier is giving money to the physician for their referral. Examples are:

- Rental amounts for space that is unnecessary or not used
- Rental amounts for time when the rented space is not in use by the supplier
- Non-exclusive occupancy of the rented portion of space

In addition, rental amount calculations should prorate rent based on the amount of space and duration of time the premises are being used. The basis for any proration should be documented and updated as necessary.

Administrative Issues

What is the Safe Harbor for space rental?

The safe harbor can protect legitimate space rental arrangements. The following are the safe harbor criteria:

- The agreement is set out in writing and signed by the parties involved, in this case the physicians and suppliers

- The agreement covers all of the premises rented by the parties for the term of the agreement and specifies the premises be covered by the agreement

- If the agreement is intended to provide the person who is leasing with access to the premises for periodic intervals of time rather than on a full-time basis for the term of the rental agreement, the rental agreement specifies exactly the schedule of such intervals, their precise length, and the exact rent for such intervals

- The term of the rental agreement is for not less than one year

- The aggregate rental charge is set in advance, is consistent with fair market value in arms-length transactions, and is not determined in a manner that takes into account the volume or value of any referrals or business otherwise generated between the parties for which payment may be made in whole or in part under Medicare or a state health care program

Arrangements that are made for office equipment or personal services of physicians' office staff can also be structured to comply with the equipment rental safe harbor and personal services and management contracts safe harbor. Specific equipment used should be identified and documented and payment limited to the prorated portion of its use. Similarly, any services provided should be documented and payment should be limited to the actual time services are performed.

Audits & Monitoring

Audit Investigation

What is the best way to prevent an audit by the federal government?

You can avoid being targeted for an audit by keeping up with changes in Medicare policy. Be sure to read all newsletters and bulletins from your carrier, attend seminars when they are offered, review remittance notices, and, most importantly, document all that you do (and bill only what is documented). Creating a compliance plan for your organization is one way to show the government that you are taking a step in the prevention of fraud and abuse in governmental health care programs, although, there is no way of escaping an audit once the audit investigation process has begun. Prevention is always the best medicine.

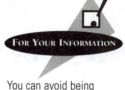

FOR YOUR INFORMATION

You can avoid being targeted for an audit by keeping up with changes in Medicare policy.

Audit Reports

What type of information should be included in an audit report?

The type of audit performed determines the content of the report. The report should include a summary of all areas reviewed. Previous or current noncompliance issues should have more detailed information, and should include comparisons with previous audit information. Most comprehensive audits should contain a variety of comparison tools. What is contained in the report should include what is effective for your practice. Some of the reporting tools are:

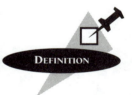

DEFINITION

Summary Report
This is a narrative description of the areas and finding of the review. This does not provide details, only a synopsis of the findings.

41

Quick Guide to Physician Fraud and Abuse Prevention

DEFINITION

Compliance Report Card
Report cards provide an overall snapshot of the current compliance issues and the effectiveness of corrective actions.

- **Summary Report** — This is a narrative description of the areas and finding of the review. This does not provide details, only a synopsis of the findings

- **Detailed Findings Section** — Areas of previous or current noncompliance that require retailed analysis and comparisons with previous audit information in order to assess the effectiveness of the corrective actions taken. In addition, any new areas of concern will require a detailed report

- **Checklists** — This is usually an information gathering tool, but should be included as supporting documentation in the compliance report. Checklists are commonly utilized to identify all the compliance elements being reviewed during the current audit so that the auditor can be sure that nothing is missed. In addition, for specific elements, a checklist is often a good tool to use when reviewing information

- **Graphs** — Graphs are useful to illustrate the effectiveness of corrective actions in targeted areas. A well-designed graphic analysis of compliance performance can provide physicians with the information they need at a glance

- **Spreadsheets** — Spreadsheets can provide pertinent information at a glance. Listed on the spreadsheet should be all information that is necessary to be able to assess the audit and/or monitoring, such as:

- Medical record number
- Date of Service
- Physician
- Physician Asst. (If available)
- ICD-9-CM diagnosis code reported
- ICD-9-CM procedural code reported
- CPT code reported
- CPT code revised
- Any explanation of changes made during the audit

Audits & Monitoring

- **Compliance Report Card** — Each area audited should be listed and the key elements assessed. Report cards provide an overall snapshot of the current compliance issues and the effectiveness of corrective actions. A report could contain:

- Areas that require continuous monitoring

- Areas where compliance elements have been met and no longer require review

- Areas of new concern

Audit Resources

What type of resources do I need to perform a coding and billing audit?

If an audit on coding and billing information is performed, the auditor should have the following resources:

- CPT book for the appropriate year of the documentation that is being audited

- ICD-9-CM book for the appropriate year of the documentation that is being audited

- HCPCS book for the appropriate year of the documentation that is being audited

- Copy of the HCFA-1500 to be billed or that has been billed

- Superbill

- Fee schedule

- EOB (Explanation of Benefits) or EOMB (Explanation of Medicare Benefits) (if it has already been billed and reimbursed by the payer)

- Organization's policies applicable to auditing and monitoring

- Any documentation supporting a payer's decision on a coding issue(s)

- Any newsletter from a credible source (e.g., AMA, HCFA, Medicare carrier, or fiscal intermediary)

- Medicare carrier bulletins

43

Quick Guide to Physician Fraud and Abuse Prevention

- Third party payer guidelines
- Copy of Correct Coding Initiative edits for time frame audited

Note: Resources are dependent on the payer and claims audited.

Audit Sample Size

How do you establish the size of your audit sample?

The sample should be large enough to provide a good representation. Minimum standards are 10-30 charts or documents per physician or 5-10 percent of all patient visits during a given time period. However, the sample size will vary according to the size of the organization and the volume of services, as well as the risk associated with each specific auditing issue.

Audit Sources

How are physicians selected for an audit?

The physician's charge pattern or practice profile is the primary source for audit selection. This computerized data is used to compare physicians with others of the same specialty in the same geographic area to determine whether their charges or levels of service are beyond the norm. Once aberrance is identified, further investigation (e.g., a focused medical review) is performed to determine its cause. Once the cause of the aberrance is determined, corrective action is taken. However, if fraudulent practices are uncovered during the course of a medical review, these cases will be referred to the carrier fraud unit for further investigation. This includes cases in which there is a history of educational contacts and denials that have been unsuccessful in correcting the physician's aberrant behavior.

The Office of the Inspector General (OIG) may also ask the carrier to audit a physician based on tips received from

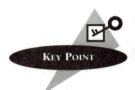

KEY POINT

The sample should be large enough to provide a good representation.

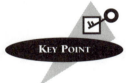

KEY POINT

The physician's charge pattern or practice profile is the primary source for audit selection.

44

hospitals, physician employees, patients, or other physicians. These individuals are known as "whistleblowers," and under the Incentive Program for Fraud and Abuse Information created under HIPAA, Medicare beneficiaries and others who report fraud and/or abuse in the Medicare program can be paid reward money if their information leads directly to the recovery of Medicare money.

Auditing an In-Office Laboratory

Who should be involved when auditing an in-house laboratory?

Because a laboratory is such a high-risk area, an employee or an outside consultant who is an expert in the field should be assigned to work with the auditing team. This clinical expert shares their knowledge throughout the course of the auditing process and will assist in clinical areas that auditors won't often look. They identify some of the more in-depth questions and help the auditors get to the information they need in regards to the areas that are being audited.

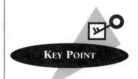

Because a laboratory is such a high-risk area, an employee or an outside consultant who is an expert in the field should be assigned to work with the auditing team.

E/M Documentation Requirements

What guidelines are available to use for auditing E/M services?

There are two sets of E/M guidelines available for use when auditing. The American Medical Association (AMA) and the Health Care Financing Administration (HCFA) have developed both of these. The first are the 1995 guidelines. They involve the history, which includes:

- Chief complaint (CC)
- History of present illness (HPI)
- Review of systems (ROS)
- Past, family, and social history (PFSH)

The physical examination includes the following body areas:

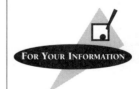

There are two sets of E/M guidelines available for use when auditing.

- Head, including face
- Neck
- Chest, including breasts and axilla
- Abdomen
- Genitalia, groin, and buttocks
- Back
- Each extremity

and/or organ systems:

- Eyes
- Ears, nose, mouth, and throat
- Cardiovascular
- Respiratory
- Gastrointestinal
- Genitourinary
- Musculoskeletal
- Skin
- Neurologic
- Psychiatric
- Hematologic/lymphatic/immunologic

Medical decision making involves:

- Number of diagnoses or management options
- Amount and/or complexity of data reviewed
- Risk of complications and/or morbidity, mortality

The second set of guidelines available for use are the 1997 guidelines. The key components of history and medical decision making are equivalent to the components in the 1995 guidelines, but the physical examination is audited differently. The guidelines use single system organ examination and a general multi-system exam table (these may be found on HCFA's or the AMA's website).

Either one of the sets of guidelines may be used to audit records, using the one that is the most beneficial to the provider.

How can I ensure that my documentation meets the E/M criteria?

One key to documenting appropriately is physician commitment to understanding the current documentation requirements and then changing their documentation habits to meet those requirements. Many physician offices purchase or develop documentation templates (both multi-system and specialty specific) to aid physicians in documenting all the essential elements of the services they provide.

Also, by using a checklist, conduct a monthly audit of a sample of each physician's charts. Review different levels of evaluation and management (E/M) services. Provide feedback to the physician as to the results of your audit, and monitor compliance. Develop an audit checklist that includes:

- The "history" components (chief complaint, history of present illness, review of systems, and past/family/social history)
- Physical examination specifications (general multi-system or single organ specialty exam)
- The three elements of medical decision making (number of diagnosis/management options, tests reviewed/ordered, and risk of complications, morbidity, or mortality)

If necessary, provide training in the E/M documentation requirements for the E/M services.

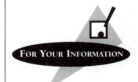

For Your Information

Many physician offices purchase or develop documentation templates to aid physicians in documenting all the essential elements of the services they provide.

Employee Performing Audit Functions

What are the advantages/disadvantages of having an audit performed by an employee of the practice?

The advantage of having an employee of the practice as auditor is that he/she is more familiar with the organization's processes, departmental organization, and the other employees and their work habits. It would take less time to become familiar with administrative and process issues. An in-house employee would also be more cost effective than outside consultants. Outside consultants usually charge a higher rate for their services. The disadvantages of having an auditor from in-house is that he/she may be more biased toward employee's work habits and not be objective. The individual may be too familiar with processes and overlook an issue(s) that an outside consultant may see as problematic.

Initial Audit

What are some of the common risk areas that should be looked at when performing an initial audit for a compliance plan?

Identifying some of the risk areas that are unique to a practice is important when auditing or reviewing documentation and/or business methods, but there are some more common issues that are recognized, such as:

- Billing for items of services not actually provided
- Providing medically unnecessary services
- Upcoding
- Outpatient service provided in connection with inpatient hospital stays (unbundling)
- Inappropriate balance billing
- Inadequate resolution of overpayments
- Computer software programs that encourage billing personnel to enter data in fields indicating services

KEY POINT

Identifying some of the risk areas that are unique to a practice is important when auditing or reviewing documentation and/or business methods.

Audits & Monitoring

were rendered though not actually performed or documented

- Failure to maintain the confidentially of information/records

- Knowing misuse of provider identification numbers, which results in improper billing

- Duplicate billing in an attempt to gain duplicate payment

- Billing for discharge in lieu of transfer

- Failure to properly use modifiers

- The organization's high volume/high dollar CPT codes

- Consistent claim denials of the same CPT and ICD-9-CM code combinations

- Unbundling of CPT codes

- Internal coding practices

- Assumption coding

- Sanctioned individuals

- Third party billing companies

Some other risk areas that are specific to physicians are:

- Critical care services

- Discharge management services

- Evaluation and management services

- Medical Necessity

- Modifier -25

- Nonphysician services

What should be included in the initial audit report?

The initial written audit report should contain a summary of the risk areas that have been identified. Along with these risk areas should be recommendations of corrective action that should take place to rectify compliance problems. This will assist in identifying how often the audits should occur for particular risk areas. It should also identify any areas in

49

Quick Guide to Physician Fraud and Abuse Prevention

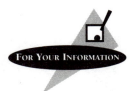

FOR YOUR INFORMATION

If a particular area of coding has been identified as problematic, it should be in the audit report detailing where the problems lie.

need of education and training, if necessary. For example, if a particular area of coding has been identified as problematic, such as Evaluation and Management, it should be in the audit report detailing where the problems lie (i.e., consultation codes) and how often the problem has occurred. Next, any regulations and guidelines from reliable sources (i.e., Medicare Carrier Manual) should be identified for further assistance.

Legal Audit

What is a legal audit?

This term refers to an internal audit review of the practice's legal liabilities based on the compliance plan it has in place, as well as to determine the revisions necessary to develop and operate an effective compliance program. This type of audit is performed by or directly supervised by legal counsel.

Monitoring Risk Areas

What are some of the areas targeted by the OIG that should be taken into consideration when monitoring risk areas?

These areas consist of:

- Billing for items or services not actually rendered
- Billing for medically unnecessary services
- Duplicate billing
- Unbundling
- Upcoding
- Incorrect modifier usage
- Incorrect code usage
- False cost reports
- Inappropriate balance billing
- Failure to refund overpayments
- Misuse of provider identification numbers
- Routine waiver of copayments

- Lack of integrity in computer systems
- Computer software programs
- Insufficient documentation
- Lost or misfiled loose sheets
- Incentives that may violate the Anti-Kickback Statute or other federal or state statutes
- Joint ventures where one party can refer Medicare or Medicaid business to the other
- Stark self-referral law
- Failure to maintain confidentiality of medical information

Monitoring Tools

What kind of tools are used to monitor the compliance program?

There are a number of ways to monitor previously identified risk areas and to potentially detect new problems. Some of these are:

- Interviews with personnel involved in management, operations, coding, billing, claim development and submission, and other related activities
- Questionnaires developed to solicit impressions from employees regarding the effectiveness of the compliance program and any new areas of concern
- Testing clinical, billing, and coding personnel on their knowledge of reimbursement coverage criteria and official coding guidelines
- Trend analyses or longitudinal studies evaluating changes in coding/billing practices or other specific areas over a given time period
- Reviews of medical and financial records and other source documents that support claims for reimbursement

Monitoring allows the compliance officer or committee to identify and review variations in an established baseline.

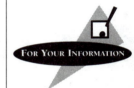

For Your Information

Ways of Monitoring Previously Identified Risk Areas
- Interviews with personnel
- Questionnaires
- Testing clinical, billing, and coding personnel
- Trend analyses or longitudinal studies
- Reviews of medical and financial records

Variations do not necessarily indicate a compliance problem. However, they should be promptly investigated to identify the cause of the variation and if the variation is a compliance issue.

Recommended Frequency of Self-Audits

How often should we perform self-auditing procedures as a part of our compliance plan?

The OIG provides very little direction on the frequency of monitoring (they state only that audits should be performed at least annually), although it should be based on the outcome of your initial audit. This will give an assessment of the level of compliance needed in specific areas of your organization and identify pertinent risk areas. The following are suggestions about when to audit:

- Annually — The entire compliance plan should be reviewed on an annual basis
- Quarterly — Targeted risk areas should be monitored every three months to assure that the problem areas are resolving or have been resolved
- Monthly — Audits should be performed monthly within each department or division that is a targeted risk area, such as billing and coding departments
- Weekly — Weekly audits should be performed if a large amount of non-compliance issues have been identified during the initial audit or during the monitoring process
- As Needed — If a potential compliance problem is uncovered, it should be addressed immediately. An audit should be performed to determine the scope of the problem. The extent of the audit will vary from problem to problem

These results should be reported to the physician or to the governing body of the organization. If you find numerous or serious errors, institute a comprehensive training program for all staff involved.

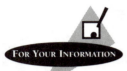

For Your Information

Frequency of Monitoring
- Annually
- Quarterly
- Monthly
- Weekly
- As Needed

Billing Policies

Balance Billing

What is balance billing?

Nonparticipating physicians who do not accept assignment on a claim may charge up to 15 percent more than the Medicare recommended amount, with the patient paying the balance out of pocket. This is known as balance billing.

Medicare regulations specifically indicate that health care professionals have two available options. One is to sign up with Medicare, which requires them to accept the Medicare payment amount as payment in full, and enables them to bill Medicare directly and receive prompt payment. Health care professionals' other option is not to participate in Medicare, which enables them to charge up to 15 percent more than the Medicare payment amount, with the patient paying the balance out of pocket when the physician chooses not to accept assignment on the claim.

Currently, federal law states that no person is liable for payment of any amount billed in excess of the limiting charge. Any health care provider who exceeds this amount must take the following actions:

- Refund to the patient the full amount collected that was above 115 percent of the Medicare allowed amount
- Reduce the outstanding balance owed for other items and services provided to the patient by the amount of the charge above the limiting charge, and refund any amount exceeding the outstanding balance

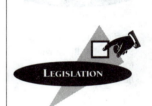

Federal law states that no person is liable for payment of any amount billed in excess of the limiting charge.

Quick Guide to Physician Fraud and Abuse Prevention

- If excess charges have not yet been collected, reduce the patient's actual charge to the Medicare approved amount

Carriers carefully screen all nonassigned claims submitted by nonparticipating providers and suppliers. If an overcharge is discovered, the provider or supplier is notified within 30 days. The provider then has 30 days to refund the overcharge to the patient or credit the patient's account.

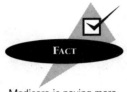

FACT

Medicare is paying more attention to those who routinely violate the balance billing regulations.

Medicare is paying more attention to those who routinely violate the balance billing regulations, especially those providers who refuse to refund money to patients. The Social Security Act Amendments of 1994 state that physicians, other practitioners, and suppliers are liable for charges that exceed the federal limiting charges for services to which they apply. A provider who repeatedly, knowingly, and willfully exceeds the limiting charges could face heavy sanctions, including extensive fines or exclusion from the Medicare program.

The Health Insurance Portability and Accountability Act of 1996 amends the civil monetary provisions of the Social Security Act by increasing the amount of the penalty for violating the balance billing limit from $2,000 to $10,000 for each item or service involved. It also increases the assessment to which a person may be subject from twice the amount to three times the amount claimed for such item or service in lieu of damages sustained by the United States or a state agency because of such a claim. In addition, the physician, other practitioner, or supplier may still be excluded from the Medicare program for up to five years.

Billing for Phone Calls

Can I bill Medicare or the patient for telephone calls?

No. These services should not be billed separately. Services provided by means of a telephone conversation between

54

Billing Policies

the physician and the patient, or between the physician and a patient's family member, are covered under the Medicare program. However, separate payment will not be made for these services because they are considered an integral component of the physician's service (e.g., evaluation and management). Medicare views telephone services as part of the pre- and post-work of a physician's service and included in the payment for those services as indicated in the Medicare Carriers Manual.

Billing Referral Services

What are the specific claim form requirements when billing for referral services?

All claims for Medicare services and items that are provided as the result of a physician's order or referral must include the referring physician's unique physician identification number (UPIN) on the HCFA-1500 claim form. This includes claims for the following:

- Parenteral and enteral nutrition
- Immunosuppressive drugs
- Diagnostic laboratory services
- Diagnostic radiology services
- Consultative services
- Durable medical equipment

Claims for any other services ordered or referred by a physician but not included on the above list must also show the UPIN of the ordering or referring physician. For example, a surgeon must complete Items 17 and 17a of the HCFA-1500 claim form when a physician refers a patient. When the ordering physician is also the performing physician, which is often true with clinical laboratory tests performed in the office, the performing physician's name and UPIN must appear in Items 17 and 17a.

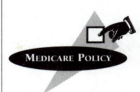

MEDICARE POLICY

All claims for Medicare services and items that are provided as the result of a physician's order or referral must include the referring physician's unique physician identification number (UPIN) on the HCFA-1500 claim form.

Care Plan Oversight and Group Practices

Can several physicians in the same group practice tally their time over the calendar month when billing for care plan oversight?

No. The care plan oversight services must be personally furnished by the physician who bills them.

If one of the members of a group practice has either significant ownership or financial interest in a home health agency (HHA), can the other physicians in the group practice sign the plan of care and bill for care plan oversight?

Yes. If the group itself has no ownership interest in the home health agency, the other members of the group can sign the plan of care and be paid for care plan oversight services.

Care Plan Oversight/Hospice

Can a volunteer medical director of a hospice bill for care plan oversight?

No. According to the Code of Federal Regulations (CFR), a volunteer within a hospice is considered an employee of the hospice. Payments to the hospice already include payment for services of the hospice physicians in establishing and overseeing the plans of care. Separate Part B payments are limited to physicians who are not affiliated with the hospice. Thus, the volunteer medical director is considered an employee of the hospice and cannot bill separately for care plan oversight under the physician fee schedule.

Care Plan Oversight Signatures

Can a primary care physician other than the physician who signed the plan of care bill for care plan oversight?

No. The physician who bills for the care plan oversight must be the same physician who signs the plan of care.

KEY POINT

The physician who bills for the care plan oversight must be the same physician who signs the plan of care.

Keep in mind that only one care plan oversight code can be billed per 30-day period per patient.

CCI Updates

If I already own a previous edition of the Correct Coding Initiative Manual, what is the benefit of owning the most recent edition?

Only by using the most recent code edit information can you be sure of receiving full and appropriate reimbursement for the medical services you provide. The additional benefit would be to avoid unbundling and decrease the likelihood of a fraud and abuse investigation. HCFA produces a completely new manual for every new version of its code edits because there are so many changes made during each revision that it would be too laborious for users to manually write them into the previous edition. Purchasing an updatable manual is recommended to avoid using outdated information.

Claim Form Signatures

If we do not include a signature in Item 12 of the HCFA-1500 claim form, what does the carrier do with the claim?

After March 1, 1996, if there is no beneficiary signature or "signature on file" indicator submitted in Item 12 of the HCFA-1500 form, the carrier returns the claim as unprocessable.

Clinical Psychologists and Clinical Social Workers and E/M Codes

Can clinical psychologists and clinical social workers bill E/M codes?

No, they bill with psychotherapy codes. Clinical psychologists may use CPT codes 90801, 90820, 90843, 90844, 90846-90857, and 90830. Clinical social workers may use CPT codes 90801, 90820, 90843, 90844, and 90846-90857.

57

Conscious Sedation

Is there a modifier or a time element that should be billed when submitting a charge for conscious sedation, code 99141?

This code includes support for the entire procedure and does not require a modifier or need an indicator of time. This includes pre and post evaluations of the patient, administration of the anesthesia, and the monitoring of cardiorespiratory functions.

The CPT book states that in order to use the conscious sedation codes, the presence of an independent trained observer to assist the physician in monitoring the patient's level of consciousness and physiological status is required. How would an independent trained observer be defined?

The American Medical Association, in accordance with the American Society of Anesthesiologists and the American Academy of Pediatrics, describes an independent trained observer: "The individual responsible for monitoring the patient should be trained in the recognition of complications associated with sedation/analgesia. In addition, at least one qualified individual capable of establishing a patient airway and positive pressure ventilation, as well as a means to summon additional assistance, should be present whenever sedation/analgesia are administered."

In addition to endoscopic procedures, we have been billing for procedure code 99141. Medicare has never paid in all of the times that we have used it. Can we bill the patient for that service since Medicare does not cover it?

No. Medicare considers code 99141 as a "bundled" code rather than a noncovered code. This means they bundle the value of the sedation into the endoscopic payment. Medicare states that all services that are necessary to perform a procedure are included in the payment for that code even if there is an independent code that exists for that service/procedure. Medicare has not paid separately for conscious sedation with an endoscopic procedure since 1991.

For noncovered services, you may bill a Medicare patient after giving them notification.

Covered Visit with Preventive Care

How would I bill a patient who was treated for an illness but also had a preventive physical on the same day?

As stated in the Medicare Carriers Manual, when the physician furnishes a Medicare beneficiary a covered visit at the same place and on the same occasion as a preventive medicine service (CPT codes 99381-99397), the covered visit will be considered in lieu of a part of the preventive medicine service of equal value to the visit. A preventive medicine service (99381-99397) is a noncovered service for Medicare. The physician may charge the beneficiary for the noncovered remainder of the service, the amount by which the physician's current established charge for the preventive medicine service exceeds his/her current established charge for the covered visit. The physician is not required to give the beneficiary written advance notice of noncoverage for the part of the visit that constitutes a routine preventive visit. However, the physician is responsible for notifying the patient in advance of his/her liability for the charges for services that are not medically necessary to treat the illness or injury.

There could be covered and noncovered procedures performed during this encounter (e.g., screening x-ray, EKG, lab tests). These would be considered individually. Those procedures that are for screening for asymptomatic conditions are considered noncovered and, therefore, no payment would be made. Those procedures ordered to diagnose or monitor a symptom, medical condition, or treatment are evaluated for medical necessity and, if covered, are paid.

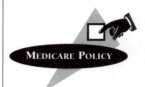

MEDICARE POLICY

A preventive medicine service is a noncovered service for Medicare.

But because these services are not covered by Medicare, they are not subject to the limiting charges. Claims for the covered portions of the service should be submitted along with noncovered portions of the service on the same claim form. If the participating provider's usual charge for procedure code 99397 (routine preventive health physical examination) is $150, the following is an example of how the HCFA-1500 form should be submitted:

- The physician determines that the covered portion of the exam is at the 99213 level, based on medical necessity. The physician's Medicare allowance for 99213 is $40.38. As per the CPT-4 manual guidelines, modifier -25 should be appended to the Office/Outpatient service code to indicate that a significant, separately identifiable E/M service was provided by the same physician on the same day as the preventive medicine service

- In Item 21, list the diagnosis code for which the covered service is rendered and follow the guide below to complete the HCFA-1500 claim form

	Item 24D *CPT/HCPCS*	*Item 24E* *Diagnosis*	*Item 24F* *Charges*
Line 1	99397	V70.0	$109.62
Line 2	99213-25	250.00	$40.38
Total			$150.00

- The physician will receive from the Medicare carrier:
$32.30 ($40.38 x 80% = $32.30)
A denial for procedure code 99397

- The physician can bill the patient for:
$109.62 (routine portion of the exam) + $8.08 (20% copayment) = $117.70

Note: All dollar amounts are fictitious and should not be used for billing purposes.

Physicians billing their claims electronically need to link the ICD-9-CM code with the appropriate procedure code. A nonparticipating physician who is not accepting assignment should use the limiting charge for 99213

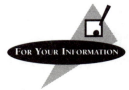

For Your Information

Physicians billing their claims electronically need to link the ICD-9-CM code with the appropriate procedure code.

Billing Policies

instead of the allowable charges used by participating physicians, and follow the rest of the example above. For both participating and nonparticipating claims, services done routinely with the complete physical examination that have not been linked to a covered medical diagnosis (for example, routine chest x-ray or routine EKG) would be denied and the patient will be responsible for those payments.

Diagnostic Coding and the Nonphysician Practitioner

Is there a regulation stating that nonphysician practitioners are required to use diagnostic codes for items and services that they render?

According to the Anti-Fraud and Abuse Provision, all nonphysician practitioners are to provide diagnostic codes for items and services rendered by the practitioner, which is already required of physicians. They should provide diagnostic or other medical information when ordering certain items or services furnished by another entity as such information is required in order for payment to be made to the entity furnishing the item of service. This requirement applies to orders for clinical laboratory tests and other diagnostic procedures, durable medical equipment, braces, and prosthetic devices.

Different Payer, Different Charge?

When Medicare is secondary for the beneficiary, can we bill the third-party payer a different charge than the one we bill to Medicare?

Medicare cannot be charged more than another payer. Electronic claims for Medicare secondary benefits must contain the necessary MSP information in the appropriate records and fields. Paper claims for Medicare secondary benefits must contain a copy of the third-party payer's explanation of benefits (EOB). The third-party payer's EOB and the Medicare claim should agree with respect to the

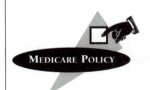

Medicare cannot be charged more than another payer.

Quick Guide to Physician Fraud and Abuse Prevention

physician's or supplier's name or code, the dates of service for the period of time over which the services were rendered, and the actual charges for the services. This information should be consistent between the Medicare claim and the third-party payer claim. However, if a claim is submitted for Medicare secondary payment and the billed charge shown on the Medicare claim differs from the billed charge shown on the third-party payer's EOB, Medicare will consider the lower amount to be the actual charge. If the third-party payment equals or exceeds the actual charge, the third-party payment will be considered payment in full. If the third-party payment is less than the actual charge, the total amount that you may collect from all sources for the service may not exceed the actual charge.

HCFA-1500 Submission Requirements

Are physicians required to complete and submit a HCFA-1500 claim form for beneficiaries? If so, are we allowed to charge the patient for this service?

The Social Security Act requires physicians and suppliers to submit Medicare Part B claims within one year for services furnished on or after Sept. 1, 1990. The Act prohibits physicians and suppliers from imposing a charge for completing and submitting a claim to Medicare. In addition, when claims for assigned services are not filed within one year of the date of service, payment is reduced by 10 percent. Physicians and suppliers who fail to submit a claim, or who impose a charge for completing a claim, are subject to sanctions, which include monetary penalties of up to $2,000 per violation and/or Medicare program exclusion.

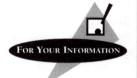

For Your Information

When claims for assigned services are not filed within one year of the date of service, payment is reduced by 10 percent.

Billing Policies

Hospital Observation During Global Surgical Period

Are hospital observation services billable during a global surgical period?

Yes, under certain circumstances, which includes:

- The hospital observation service meets the criteria needed to justify billing it with CPT modifiers -24 (unrelated evaluation and management service by the same physician during a postoperative period), -25 (significant, identifiable E/M service by the same physician on the same day of procedure or other service), or -57 (decision for major surgery)

- The hospital observation service furnished by the surgeon meets all of the criteria for the hospital observation code billed

If Item 20 Is Blank

What will happen if Item 20 of the HCFA-1500 form is left blank on a claim with procedure codes that are possibly purchased services?

After March 1, 1996, those line items that are diagnostic tests subject to the purchase price limitation are rejected by the carrier as unprocessable if Item 20 is left blank.

Incident To/Leased Nonphysicians

Can we bill "incident to" services provided by a leased nonphysician employee?

Nonphysician personnel performing an incident to service may be part-time, full-time, or leased employees of the supervising physician, physician group, or the legal entity that employs the physician who provides the supervision.

A leased employee is a nonphysician working under a written employee leasing agreement which provides that:

- The nonphysician, although employed by the leasing company, provides services as the leased employee of the physician or other entity
- The physician or other entity exercises control over all actions taken by the leased employee with regard to the rendering of medical services to the same extent as the physician or other entity would exercise such control if the leased employee were directly employed by the physician or other entity

In order to satisfy the "incident to" employment requirement, the nonphysician (whether leased or directly employed) must be considered an employee of the supervising physician or other entity under the common law test of an employer/employee relationship specified in the Social Security Act and the Retirement and Survivors Insurance program, which is part of the Social Security Program Operations Manual System.

Services provided by auxiliary personnel not employed by the physician, physician group, or other legal entity — even if provided on the physician's order or included in the physician's bill — are not covered as incident to a physician's service since the law requires that the services be of kinds commonly furnished in physicians' offices and commonly either rendered without charge or included in physicians' bills. As with the physician's personal professional services, the patient's financial liability for the incidental services is to the physician, physician group, or other legal entity. Therefore, the incidental service must represent an expense incurred by the physician, physician group, or other legal entity responsible for providing the professional service.

This does not mean, however, that to be considered "incident to" each occasion of service by a nonphysician need also always be the occasion of the actual performance of a personal professional service by the physician. Such a service could be considered to be "incident to" when furnished during a course of treatment where the physician performs an initial service and subsequent services of a

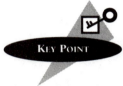

Key Point

In order to satisfy the "incident to" employment requirement, the nonphysician must be considered an employee of the supervising physician or other entity under the common law test of an employer/employee relationship specified in the Social Security Act.

frequency that reflects his active participation in and management of the course of treatment. (However, the direct supervision requirement must still be met with respect to every nonphysician service.)

Commonly furnished services are those customarily considered incident to physicians' personal services in the office or physician-directed clinic setting. The requirement could not be considered to be met where services are of a type not considered medically appropriate to provide in the office setting.

If auxiliary personnel perform services outside the office setting — in a patient's home or in an institution, for instance — their services are covered incident to a physician's services only if there is direct personal supervision by the physician. For example, if a nurse accompanies the physician on house calls and administers an injection, the nurse's services are covered; if the same nurse makes the calls alone and administers the injection, the services are not covered (even when billed by the physician) since the physician is not providing direct personal supervision. Additionally, the availability of the physician by telephone and the presence of the physician somewhere in the institution does not constitute direct personal supervision. Services provided by auxiliary personnel in an institution (e.g., hospital, skilled nursing facility, nursing or convalescent home) present a special problem in determining whether direct physician supervision exists.

Services provided by auxiliary personnel not in the employ of the physician, even if provided on the physician's order or included in the physician's bill (e.g., an independently practicing therapist who forwards his/her bill to the referring physician for inclusion in the physician's statement of services), are not covered as incident to a physician's services since the law requires that the services be of kinds commonly furnished in physicians' offices and commonly either rendered without charge or included in physicians' bills. As with the physician's personal

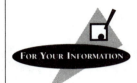

For Your Information

Commonly furnished services are those customarily considered incident to physicians' personal services in the office or physician-directed clinic setting.

professional service, the patient's financial liability for the incidental services is to the physician. Therefore, the incidental service must represent an expense incurred by the physician in his/her professional practice.

In addition to coverage being available for the services of such nonphysician personnel as nurses, technicians, and therapists when furnished incident to the professional services of a physician, a physician may also have the services of certain nonphysician practitioners who have been licensed by the state under various programs to assist or act in the place of the physician, such as certified nurse midwives, certified registered nurse anesthetists, clinical psychologists, clinical social workers, physician assistants, nurse practitioners, and clinical nurse specialists.

Services performed by these nonphysician practitioners incident to a physician's professional services include not only services ordinarily rendered by a physician's office staff person (e.g., medical services, such as taking blood pressures and temperatures, injections, and changing dressings) but also services ordinarily performed by the physician himself/herself, such as minor surgery, setting casts or simple fractures, x-ray interpretations, and other activities that involve evaluation or treatment of a patient's condition.

A nonphysician practitioner such as a physician assistant or nurse practitioner may be licensed under state law to perform a specific medical procedure and may be able to perform the procedure without physician supervision and have the service separately covered and paid for by Medicare as a physician assistant's or nurse practitioner's service. However, in order to have that same service covered as incident to, it must be performed under the direct personal supervision of the physician as an integral part of the physician's personal in-office service. This does not mean that each occasion of incidental service performed by a nonphysician practitioner must always be the occasion of a service actually rendered by the physician. It does mean that there must have been direct,

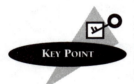

KEY POINT

Services performed by nonphysician practitioners incident to a physician's professional services include not only services ordinarily rendered by a physician's office staff person but also services ordinarily performed by the physician himself/herself.

personal, professional service furnished by the physician to initiate the course of treatment of which the service being performed by the nonphysician practitioner is an incidental part, and there must be subsequent services by the physician of a frequency that reflects his/her continuing active participation in the management of the course of treatment.

Injections

Can an injection and an E/M code be billed on the same day of service?

If an injection, coded with CPT codes 90782, 90783, 90784, or 90788, was given and no E/M service was provided, only the code for the injection should be reported. Code 99211 should not be billed for a visit if the only purpose for the visit was to receive the injection. The drug used should be billed with an "J" code.

If an E/M service is provided on the same day, the injection is considered part of the service and will not be paid separately.

In-Office Oral Medications

Can I bill for oral medications given in the office?

The Medicare Carriers Manual states that drugs that are self-administered are not covered by Medicare Part B unless the statute provides for such coverage. The self-administered drugs that are covered under the statute are drugs with blood clotting factors, drugs used in immunosuppressive therapy, erythropoietin for dialysis patients, and certain oral anti-cancer drugs.

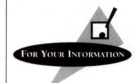

For Your Information

If an E/M service is provided on the same day, the injection is considered part of the service and will not be paid separately.

Quick Guide to Physician Fraud and Abuse Prevention

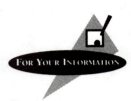

For Your Information

There are some procedures for which separate payment for a surgical tray is allowed.

In-Office Supplies

Can I bill Medicare for supplies used when procedures are performed in my office?

Under the Medicare fee schedule, the cost of supplies used to perform surgical procedures in the office — usually referred to as the "surgical tray" — is included in the practice expense portion of most procedures' relative values. However, there are some procedures for which separate payment for a surgical tray is allowed. It is important to know which procedures these are so that the tray can be separately billed and reimbursement can be obtained.

When Medicare reimburses separately for a surgical tray, it does so based on a relative value of .52, which yields a payment of approximately $19.04 (reimbursement will differ depending on the physician's geographic location).

For services rendered to Medicare patients, physician office staff may not use CPT code 99070 (miscellaneous supply) to bill supplies separately, but usually commercial payers will accept that code (check with individual payers for billing guidelines).

The procedure codes listed below are those for which Medicare will reimburse separately for a surgical tray when the procedure is performed in the physician's office.

19101	19120	19125	19126	20200	20205
20220	20225	20240	25111	28290	28292
28293	28294	28296	28297	28298	28299
32000	37609	38500	43200	43202	43220
43226	43234	43235	43239	43245	43247
43249	43250	43251	43458	45378	45379
45380	45382	45383	45384	45385	49080
49081	52005	52007	52010	52204	52214
52224	52234	52235	52240	52250	52260
52270	52275	52276	52277	52282	52283
52290	52300	52301	52305	52310	52315
57520	57522	58120	62270	85095	85102
96440	96445	96450			

Billing Policies

To obtain reimbursement for the surgical tray, HCPCS Level II code A4550 should be reported in conjunction with the code for the procedure performed.

There are additional procedures for which Medicare will allow specific supplies to be billed in addition to the procedure. The following are the codes for the procedures and the associated supply code to be billed:

Procedure Code	Specific Supply	
36533	A4300	Implantable access catheter (venous, arterial, epidural, or peritoneal), external access
68761	A4263	Permanent, long-term, nondissolvable lacrimal duct implant, each
95028	G0025	Collagen skin test

In some instances, Medicare will also allow the billing of the following supplies:

A4565	Slings
A4570	Splints
A4572	Rib belt
A4580*	Casting supplies
A4590	Special casting materials, Hexcelite and light cast
J codes	Drugs
L4350-L4380	Pneumatic splint (air cast or equal)

Unna boots are considered a dressing — not casting — and are not paid separately.

In addition, if the supply is a pharmaceutical or radiopharmaceutical imaging agent (including codes A4641-A4647); pharmacologic stressing agent (code J1245), or therapeutic radionuclide (CPT code 79900), the procedure performed must be one of the following in order for the supply to be billable:

- Diagnostic radiologic procedures (including diagnostic nuclear medicine) requiring pharmaceutical or

Quick Guide to Physician Fraud and Abuse Prevention

- radiopharmaceutical contrast media and/or pharmacological stressing agent
- Other diagnostic tests requiring a pharmacological stressing agent
- Clinical brachytherapy procedures (other than remote afterloading high intensity brachytherapy procedures (CPT code 77781-77784) for which the expendable source is included in the technical component of the relative value units)
- Therapeutic nuclear medicine procedures

Surgical dressings are not separately payable under the Medicare program.

These codes include A4190 (transparent film), A4200 (elastic gauze), A4203 (nonelastic gauze), A4204 (absorptive dressings) and A4205 (nonabsorptive dressings).

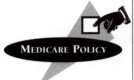

Medicare Policy

Surgical dressings are not separately payable under the Medicare program.

Item 9 and Nonparticipating Providers

The HCFA-1500 claim form instructions state that Item 9 should be completed only by participating providers. What will happen if a nonparticipating provider completes this information?

It could cause a delay in the processing of your claims. Typically a message will appear on your explanation of medical benefits (EOMB) stating that the carrier does not cross over claims for nonparticipating providers.

Leaving Blanks on the HCFA-1500 Claim Form

If information is included on the HCFA-1500 form in Items that the instructions indicate to leave blank, will it cause any problems with the processing of our claims?

Having information in these items should not cause problems in the processing of your claims, however the information will not be recognized or processed.

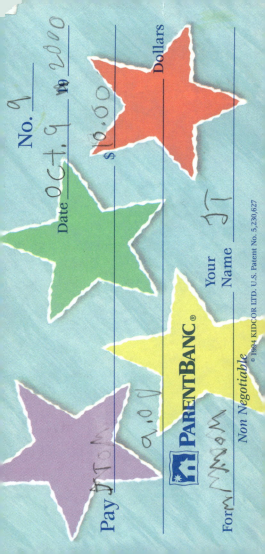

Billing Policies

Limited Licensed Practitioners

Should limited licensed practitioners (LLPs) be restricted to certain evaluation and management codes?

There are no absolute restrictions in the use of higher level codes by LLPs. However, the requirements for billing higher level codes must be met and may be dependent on the state laws governing the scope of practice of LLPs.

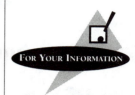

FOR YOUR INFORMATION

There are no absolute restrictions in the use of higher level codes by LLPs.

Linking Requirement

Could you clarify the linking requirement on the HCFA-1500 claim form?

Linking is the process by which specific ICD-9-CM diagnosis codes are associated with specific CPT/HCPCS codes listed in Item 24d. Item 24e contains the reference numbers that "link" the two codes. Medicare requires this linkage on the HCFA-1500 claim form. Other third-party payers also require that Item 24e be completed.

At least one valid diagnosis code must be related to each procedure or service reported on the claim in Item 24d. It is not unusual for a procedure or service to relate to several or all of the diagnosis codes listed. To ensure billing accuracy, the link must be provided between the procedure and the ICD-9-CM diagnosis code at the time of billing. If the procedures and services (Item 24d) are not linked to valid ICD-9-CM diagnosis codes, the claim will be denied. If there is a pattern of ICD-9-CM coding errors and/or noncompliance with the linking requirement, this may flag your practice for an audit.

Item 24e is used to enter all of the reference numbers for the diagnosis or diagnoses that pertain to the dates of service and specific procedure code reported on each line in Items 24a-24d (Procedures, Services, or Supplies).

A reference code number (1, 2, 3, or 4), shown in Item 21 next to each of four spaces for the ICD-9-CM codes, must

Quick Guide to Physician Fraud and Abuse Prevention

correlate with the most appropriate code for the specific service entered on the detail lines (Items 24a-24d).

Up to four codes may be reported to accurately describe the reason for the service. The first code listed should identify the condition chiefly responsible for the service. Additional codes describing coexisting conditions should follow.

For Medicare, do not provide a narrative description of the diagnosis on the billing form in this item. Medicare allows only one reference per line item. When multiple services are performed, the primary reference number (1, 2, 3, or 4) for each service is entered. Other third-party payers may allow more than one reference number to be entered in this field.

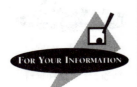

For Your Information

For Medicare, do not provide a narrative description of the diagnosis on the billing form.

Misleading Suppliers' Advice

If an individual comes to a physician's office selling supplies and gives the physician advice on coding claims for those supplies and related services, would the physician have any responsibility if that billing advice turns out to be a misrepresentation or billing for services not rendered?

Yes. As long as these supplies and services are billed using the physician's Medicare provider number, regardless of the source of advice, the physician is considered fully responsible. This is because the filing of the claim denotes the physician's certification that the services reported were actually rendered and/or that the supplies billed were provided or used. In order to avoid such situations, the physician should make every effort to verify that any billing advice he/she is given is correct before following it.

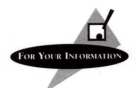

For Your Information

The physician should make every effort to verify that any billing advice he/she is given is correct before following it.

Billing Policies

Nursing Facility Admissions and Other Outpatient Service Codes

Can an office, outpatient, or emergency department visit be billed on the same day as a nursing facility admission?

No. The evaluation and management services should be bundled together for the same dates of service when the services are provided by the same physician.

Office Visits for Pneumococcal Pneumonia Vaccine (PPV)

If a physician sees a beneficiary for the sole purpose of administering PPV, may he/she routinely bill for an office visit?

No. However, if a patient actually receives other services constituting an evaluation and management service for a different problem or symptom, the physician may bill for a visit and Medicare will pay for the visit if it is reasonable and medically necessary.

Plan of Care on File

Is a "plan of care on file" statement still needed in Item 19 of the HCFA-1500 claim form for occupational and physical therapy claims?

No. However, the attending physician's UPIN and the date the patient was last seen must still be submitted.

Postoperative Care/Second Physician

How do we bill for postoperative care performed by a cardiologist following cardiac surgery performed by a cardiovascular surgeon? This is a very common occurrence for our practice.

Payment for postoperative care is typically included in the payment for the global surgery package. The following are

73

the payment guidelines for postoperative care when performed by two physicians:

- The services of the cardiologist are for an underlying condition or medical complication, they should be paid by Medicare as medically necessary concurrent care, using evaluation and management (E/M) codes. Be sure to report on the claim the specific diagnosis code that identifies the underlying condition or medical complication that necessitated the cardiologist's services. Documentation may be requested by the payer to substantiate the medical necessity of the concurrent care

- The services of the cardiologist are not for a separate medical condition and are not medically necessary, they would be denied by Medicare as not covered since these services are a part of the global surgical payment to the cardiovascular surgeon

- The cardiologist should not bill using modifier -55 (postoperative management only) unless there is a transfer of care from the surgeon. For transfer of care there must be an agreement between the physicians for the postoperative care to be split. The agreement may be in the form of a letter or an annotation in the discharge summary/hospital record or ASC record. The receiving physician (cardiologist) uses the surgical procedure code with a -55 modifier and the date of assumed care in Item 19 of the HCFA-1500 claim form. The receiving physician cannot bill for any part of the service included in a global period until he/she has provided at least one service. In this case, the surgeon would submit his/her claim with the appropriate procedure code with modifier -54 (surgical care only) and the date care was relinquished in Item 19 of the HCFA-1500 claim form

Billing Policies

Prolonged Services

Can you bill prolonged services codes alone?

No. All prolonged service codes should be billed along with an E/M code in order for payment to be made. The following is a list of codes that should be billed:

- Code 99354 should be billed with E/M codes 99201-99205, 99212-99215, or 99241-99245
- Code 99355 should be billed with 99354 and E/M codes 99201-99205, 99212-99215, or 99241-99245
- Code 99356 should be billed with E/M codes 99221-99223, 99231-99233, 99251-99255, 99261-99263, 99301-99303, or 99311-99313
- Code 99357 should be billed with 99356 and E/M codes 99221-99223, 99231-99233, 99251-99255, 99261-99263, 99301-99303, or 99311-99313

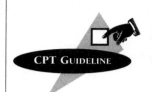

All prolonged service codes should be billed along with an E/M code in order for payment to be made.

What are the requirements for using prolonged services codes in addition to the E/M code?

Only the duration of direct face-to-face contact between the physician and the patient (whether the service was continuous or not) beyond the typical time of the visit code billed will be used to determine whether prolonged services can also be billed and to determine which prolonged services codes are allowable. To use prolonged office service codes, time spent by office staff with the patient, or time the patient remains unaccompanied in the office cannot be billed. For prolonged hospital services, time spent waiting for test results, for changes in the patient's condition, for end of a therapy, or for use of facilities cannot be billed as prolonged services.

Do I need to send documentation to Medicare to support the use of a prolonged service code?

No. Medicare does not require documentation to accompany the bill for prolonged services unless the physician has been targeted for medical review. The medical record must contain the duration and content of the E/M

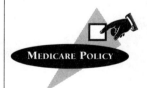

Medicare does not require documentation to accompany the bill for prolonged services unless the physician has been targeted for medical review.

75

Quick Guide to Physician Fraud and Abuse Prevention

service billed and demonstrate that the physician personally furnished at least 30 additional minutes of direct service after the typical time of the E/M service.

Signature Required

What will be done with claims that do not have a provider signature in Item 31 of the HCFA-1500 form?

After March 1, 1996, if there is no provider signature submitted in Item 31, the claim will be returned as unprocessable.

Stand-By Services

Are "stand-by" services billable to Medicare?

Part B benefits cannot be provided for time spent by the surgeon standing by in case surgical expertise is required since this service is excluded by Medicare law. Medicare patients may not be billed by the physician for this service, either.

Physician stand-by services are covered as inpatient hospital services, not as physician services, since standing by is not a service to the patient. Payment for this service is included in the payment made to the hospital for other general services necessary for the provision of quality care.

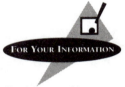

For Your Information

Physician stand-by services are covered as inpatient hospital services.

Written Billing Policies

Do I need written policies for billing and claims processing?

A written billing and claims processing policy is not required by law, but it can serve to protect the practice in the event of an investigation.

With the increase in audit investigations, the need for up-to-date billing policies is more crucial than ever in defending against fraud and abuse accusations. An up-to-date, well-drafted policy and procedure manual containing the practice's basic policies can reduce confusion within the

Billing Policies

practice and often provide an effective defense evidence as to the practice's intent and expectations concerning billing.

For these reasons, more and more physicians are using policy and procedure manuals to help establish uniform policies, as well as training tools for new employees.

Coding Policies

Assumption Coding

What is assumption coding?

Assumption coding is where documentation may be illegible or unclear and the coder assumes what is written without questioning the health care provider. The coder then applies a code that may be incorrect for a service or procedure. It is important that there is open communication with the physician if there is a question of what is written or transcribed and the coder should question the health care provider for clarification. The individual who performs coding duties should fully understand the ramifications of assumptive coding and have the education and/or experience to prevent miscoding due to assumption coding.

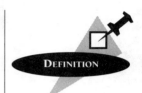

DEFINITION

Assumption coding is where documentation may be illegible or unclear and the coder assumes what is written without questioning the health care provider.

Bundling Lesion Excision and Repair Codes

Can the excision of a lesion and a repair code be billed together?

According to the Medicare Carriers Manual, it is dependent on if the lesion is benign or malignant and if the repair is simple, intermediate, or complex. Simple repairs (CPT codes 12001-12018) should not be reported with CPT codes 11400-11446 (excision of benign lesions) or 11600-11646 (excision of malignant lesions). CPT codes 11400, 11420, and 11440 include a simple, intermediate, or complex repair, and should not be coded separately. If an intermediate (CPT codes 12031-12057) or complex repair (CPT codes 13100-13153) is performed in addition to codes 11406 and 11421-11426 (excision of benign

Quick Guide to Physician Fraud and Abuse Prevention

lesion(s)) or codes 11600-11646, both the excision code and the repair code may be reported.

CCI's Effect on Claims

What is the CCI and how does it affect my claims?

The CCI is HCFA's National Correct Coding Initiative, which became effective on Jan. 1, 1996. Under the CCI, HCFA has developed general policies that define coding principles and comprehensive edits that apply to procedures and service codes.

Since the installation of the correct coding edits into the claims processing system, Medicare uses to detect inappropriate coding practices, Medicare rejections have multiplied. With the passage of the Health Insurance Portability and Accountability Act of 1996, correct coding practices are no longer optional but mandatory.

Most Medicare carriers had already included in their claims processing systems various computerized edits to detect improper coding of procedures. Many of these were designed to detect "fragmentation," the separate coding of the component parts of a procedure when a single code encompassing the entire procedure should have been used.

Unfortunately, there was no consistency or uniformity among carriers in the usage of the correct coding edits for two reasons. First, individual carriers had used their own discretion in establishing priorities and direction of efforts to standardize coding methodologies. Secondly, data availability and analysis expertise necessary for the identification of the component parts of a comprehensive procedure are not easily accessible.

The greatest impact on the provider from the CCI edits has been to those who have a misunderstanding of appropriate code selection. Most of the edits are focused on unbundling and the coding of mutually exclusive procedures.

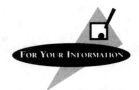

FOR YOUR INFORMATION

Most Medicare carriers had already included in their claims processing systems various computerized edits to detect improper coding of procedures.

Coding Policies

Consultations vs. Visits

I feel, as an orthopaedic surgeon, that all my initial patient visits are consultations. Would billing them as such be a problem?

Yes, if the visit does not meet the criteria for a consultation. According to the Medicare Carriers Manual, a consultation is generally considered to be different from a visit because:

- It is done at the request of a referring physician (unless it is a patient-generated confirmatory consultation)

- The consultant prepares a report of his/her findings, which are provided to the referring physician for the referring physician's use in treatment of the patient

A consultant may initiate diagnostic and/or therapeutic services. However, when the referring physician orally or in writing transfers responsibility of treatment at the time of the request for the consultation or referral, the receiving physician may not bill a consultation but should bill this as an initial office visit.

CPO Requirement

Can the time an attending physician spends discussing, with his/her nurse, conversations the nurse had with the home health agency count toward the 30-minute requirement of care plan oversight?

No. Time spent with the nurse does not count toward the 30-minute threshold. However, the time the physician spends working on the care plan, after the nurse has conveyed the pertinent information, is countable toward the 30 minutes.

Quick Guide to Physician Fraud and Abuse Prevention

CPO/Two Physicians

Can the time another physician spends working on the patient's care with the attending physician who actually signed the care plan be counted toward the 30-minute requirement of care plan oversight?

No. Only the time the attending physician spends on care plan oversight is countable. The time spent by other physicians is not countable toward the 30-minute requirement. Payment for care plan oversight is for the time spent by one physician — the physician providing the service.

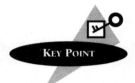

Payment for care plan oversight is for the time spent by one physician — the physician providing the service.

Critical Care

Can I code critical care services if they were provided in the office or emergency department and paid by Medicare?

Payment may be made for critical care services provided in any location as long as the care meets the definition of critical care.

A definition of critical care is direct delivery by a physician of medical care for a critically ill or injured patient. It involves decision making of high complexity to assess, manipulate, and support circulatory, central nervous system failure, circulatory failure, shock-like conditions, renal, hepatic, metabolic or respiratory failure, postoperative complications, overwhelming infection, or other vital systems functions to prevent or treat single or multiple vital organ system failure.

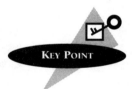

Payment may be made for critical care services provided in any location as long as the care meets the definition of critical care.

What procedure codes are bundled into critical care codes 99291 and 99292 if performed by the same physician on the same date of service?

The following codes are bundled into 99291 and 99292 when performed by the same physician on the same date of service according to Medicare:

82

36000	36410	36415	36600	71010	71015
71020	91105	92953	93561	93562	94656
94657	94660	94662	94762	99090	G0001

Any service not on this list performed in addition to codes 99291 and 99292 may be coded separately.

How many days may critical care be billed?

Critical care is not restricted to a fixed number of days. As long as the criteria for critical care are met and the services are reasonable and necessary to treat illness or injury, Medicare will reimburse for critical care services. However, claims for seemingly improbably amounts of critical care on the same date of service may be subjected to review to determine if the physician has filed a false claim.

Cystourethroscopy and Ureteral Catheterization

If both ureters are examined and catheterized during a cystourethroscopy, how is that reported?

Code 52005 should only be reported once, even if both ureters are catheterized. The work RVUs that are given to this procedure have already taken into account that it may be necessary to examine and catheterize one or both ureters. The catheterization is not reportable, as well as the examination of both ureters by appending modifier -50 or -51 to the first or an additional 52005 code.

Dictation and Time

If I'm dictating records in front of the patient, can this be considered in the time category?

Yes, it can be considered in the overall time spent with the patient, but remember that most Evaluation and Management codes are selected on the basis of time only when counseling and/or coordination of care dominates the encounter (i.e., constitutes 50 percent or more of the visit). Dictation time does not count as counseling or coordination of care.

KEY POINT

Dictation time does not count as counseling or coordination of care.

E/M Based on Time

What criteria must be met and what documentation do I need when I am coding a visit based on "time" alone for an encounter spent primarily (over 50 percent) counseling the patient?

As per the Medicare Carriers Manual, when counseling and/or coordination of care takes up more than 50 percent of the face-to-face physician/patient encounter (or the floor time in the case of inpatient services), time is the key or controlling factor in selecting the level of service. The code selection is based on the total time of the face-to-face encounter or floor time, not just the counseling time. The medical record must be documented in sufficient detail to justify the selection of the specific code if time is the basis for the selection of the code.

In the office or other outpatient setting, counseling and/or coordination of care must be provided in the presence of the patient if the time spent providing those services is used to determine the level of service reported. Face-to-face time refers to the physician's time with the patient only. Counseling by other staff is not considered to be part of the face-to-face physician/patient encounter time. Therefore, any time spent by the other staff is not considered in selecting the appropriate level of service. The code used depends upon the physician service provided.

In an inpatient setting, the counseling and/or coordination of care must be provided at the bedside or on the patient's hospital floor or unit. Time spent counseling the patient or coordinating the patient's care after the patient has left the office or the physician has left the patient's floor or begun to care for another patient on the floor is not considered when selecting the level of service to be reported.

The duration of counseling or coordination of care that is provided face-to-face or on the floor may be estimated, but that estimate, along with the total duration of the visit, must be recorded in the medical record when time is used

Key Point

Time spent counseling the patient or coordinating the patient's care after the patient has left the office or the physician has left the patient's floor or begun to care for another patient on the floor is not considered when selecting the level of service to be reported.

Coding Policies

for the selection of a level of service that involves predominately coordination of care or counseling.

E/M: New vs. Established Patient

If a physician changes practices and sees a patient that he/she had seen at the old practice at the new practice, would that patient be a new or established patient?

The patient would be an established patient. The definition of a new patient is an individual who has not received any professional services from the physician within the past three years. The site of the service is not of significance, in this case.

From Observation to Inpatient Status

If the physician admits a patient to observation but the patient's condition worsens and the physician then admits the patient as an inpatient, can we bill two separate visits?

No. You cannot bill an initial observation care code for services on the date that the physician admits the patient to inpatient status. The initial hospital visit evaluation and management codes include all services provided to the patient on the date of admission by that physician, regardless of the site of service, as stated in the Medicare Carriers Manual.

KEY POINT

You cannot bill an initial observation care code for services on the date that the physician admits the patient to inpatient status.

Hospital Admissions

If I see a patient in my office and admit him or her to the hospital on the same day, can I code each as a separate visit?

No. The Medicare Carriers Manual specifically indicates that all services provided by the physician in conjunction with that admission are considered part of the initial hospital care when performed on the same date as the admission. This also corresponds with the AMA's CPT manual guidelines for hospital inpatient services.

Immunizations

What are "combination" vaccines?

Combination vaccines are made of two or more different vaccines in a single dosage. These vaccines describe one injection of the combination vaccine and should be coded as such. All the components (e.g., Tetanus and diphtheria toxoids (Td)) that are included in the one injection should not be coded separately.

Incomplete Colonoscopy

How do we code an incomplete colonoscopy?

When the physician attempts to perform a colonoscopy, but is unable to extend the scope beyond the splenic flexure, the procedure is considered to be an incomplete or failed colonoscopy. When a failed colonoscopy is performed it should be reported with 45378, and modifier -53 should be attached to indicate the terminated diagnostic procedure. Payment for the terminated procedure will be made by the carrier, based on the value of 45330 for a flexible sigmoidoscopy.

Interpretation of Purified Protein Derivative of Tuberculin (PPD)

How is the interpretation of a PPD test coded?

The interpretation of a PPD test is considered to be a part of the medical decision making component of an evaluation and management service and should not be reported separately.

Modifier -80

Can modifier -80 (assistant surgeon) be used for nonphysicians who assist at surgery?

Modifier -80 is used for physicians only and not for non-MD/DO surgical assistants. However, modifier -AS, a HCPCS Level II, may be used when a physician assistant,

KEY POINT

The interpretation of a PPD test is considered to be a part of the medical decision making component of an evaluation and management service.

Coding Policies

nurse practitioner, or clinical nurse specialist is used for an assistant at surgery.

"Mutually Exclusive" Policy

What does "mutually exclusive" mean in the correct coding policies?

Codes are considered to be mutually exclusive if they represent services or procedures that should not or could not reasonably have been performed during the same encounter. The phrase also refers to situations where two procedures representing two different methods to accomplish the same therapeutic result may have been employed and only the successful procedure (method) should be reported. "Initial" and "subsequent" services are also considered mutually exclusive, since the physician either provided one or the other. When mutually exclusive codes are billed together, Medicare reimburses the lowest value service and the physician is not allowed to submit a corrected billing or receive additional payment.

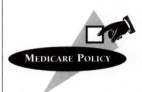

MEDICARE POLICY

When mutually exclusive codes are billed together, Medicare reimburses the lowest value service and the physician is not allowed to submit a corrected billing or receive additional payment.

Observation Unit Visits

If we are not the admitting physician and we see a patient in the observation unit at the hospital, do we code these services as an inpatient visit?

As stated in the Medicare Carriers Manual, all physicians other than the admitting physician who see the patient while he/she is in the observation unit of the hospital must code these services using the office and other outpatient service codes or outpatient consultation codes, as appropriate, when they provide services to the patient.

For example, if an internist admits a patient to observation and asks an allergist for a consultation on the patient's condition, only the internist may bill the initial observation care code. The allergist must bill using the outpatient consultation code that best represents the services he/she

87

provided. The allergist cannot bill an inpatient consultation since the patient was not a hospital inpatient.

Previous History and Physical

If the patient comes in for a follow-up visit, let's say six months after the initial visit, so the physician can see how he/she is doing, can we use the history and physical documentation obtained six months before in coding the follow-up visit?

You may not use the previous physical documentation for the current visit but you may use the review of systems (ROS) and the past, family, and social (PFS) history information taken at an earlier date. However, to do this you must direct the reviewer to the earlier date and document any update to the previous history.

If the physician needed to update this information, the updating of the information would be considered in selecting a code. Additionally, if the physician had to review previous information to make a treatment decision, this information would impact the medical decision-making component of code selection. The fact that a history was taken at a previous encounter, however, has no impact on code selection for the current encounter.

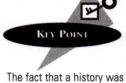

KEY POINT

The fact that a history was taken at a previous encounter, has no impact on code selection for the current encounter.

Same-Day E/M Services

How do we code a critical care service, emergency room service, or hospital visit provided on the same day?

The following HCFA guidelines apply to critical care and other E/M visits billed on the same date of service:

- If critical care is required upon presentation to the emergency department, only critical care codes (99291-99292) may be reported. Emergency department codes will not be paid for the same day

- If there is a hospital visit early in the day and at that time the patient does not require critical care, but the patient requires critical care later in the day, both critical care and a hospital visit may be paid. The use of modifier -25 will assist in identifying the services as separately identifiable on the claim

- Documentation must be submitted when critical care is billed on the same day as other E/M services

Be sure to link the specific diagnosis codes to each of the E/M services on the claim to facilitate claims processing.

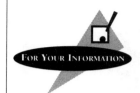

Documentation must be submitted when critical care is billed on the same day as other E/M services.

Sentinel Node Biopsy

What is a sentinel node biopsy and how is it coded?

A sentinel node biopsy is a surgical procedure that excises the first lymph node in a chain of lymph nodes. This first lymph node receives lymphatic fluid that usually drains from the site of the tumor. Because many cancer growths extend inevitably to the lymphatic system where cancer cells may become entrapped in a lymph node(s), the biopsy of the first lymph node may identify the presence or absence of a cancerous tumor. This may provide important information to the physician such as:

- Staging information to determine treatment options, prognosis, and survival
- The possible presence of metastasis

A sentinel node biopsy is coded with one of the following codes:

38500   38505   38510   38520   38525   38530   38542

Code selection depends on the location of the lymph node. If an injection procedure is performed to identify the site of the sentinel node, report 38792, or for lymph node imaging, report 78195.

Two Admission Visits

Should we code two initial hospital admission visits if two different MDs or DOs are involved in the same admission?

No. As the guidelines in the AMA's CPT manual state, initial hospital care codes (99221-99223) are used to report the first hospital inpatient encounter with the patient by the admitting physician. Only one MD or DO would be considered to be the admitting physician and be eligible to use the initial hospital care codes. The other would bill consultation services or subsequent hospital care, as appropriate.

Two Visits, Same Day

Would I use two separate codes if I treated the same patient in my office twice on the same day?

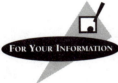

For Your Information

If the visits were for a related condition, you would only code one office visit with the combined appropriate level of service.

If the visits were for a related condition, you would only code one office visit with the combined appropriate level of service. Only if the visits were for unrelated problems that could not be treated during the same encounter could they be separately coded, according to the Medicare Carriers Manual. For example, an office visit for a blood pressure check, followed five hours later by a visit for the evaluation of leg pain following an accident could be coded separately. Be sure, though, that when you submit such a claim that the correct diagnosis codes are linked to the different E/M codes to demonstrate that they were separately identifiable visits. In addition, be sure the documentation in the medical record clearly supports the separately identifiable circumstances and diagnostic conditions.

"Unbundling" Defined

What is unbundling?

Unbundling is a type of incorrect coding. It is essentially the billing of multiple procedure codes for a group of procedures that are covered by a single, comprehensive code. There are two types of incorrect coding —

Coding Policies

intentional and unintentional. Unintentional incorrect coding results from a misunderstanding of coding. Intentional incorrect coding is used by providers to manipulate coding in order to maximize payment.

Examples of unbundling include the following:

- Fragmenting one service into component parts and coding each component part as if it were a separate service
- Reporting separate codes for related services when one comprehensive code includes all related services
- Breaking out bilateral procedures when one code is appropriate
- Downcoding a service in order to use an additional code when one higher level, more comprehensive code is appropriate
- Separating a surgical approach from a major surgical service

Using ED History

If a physician (e.g., an internist), upon admitting a patient to the hospital, wants to use the data (form) used by the emergency department physician to avoid the repetitive effort of collecting patient history information, is it acceptable to use the emergency department physician's data in the admitting physician's selection of procedure code?

If the emergency department physician has taken and reviewed the history as part of his/her evaluation and management of the patient, the admitting physician will, of course, need to review this information in his/her evaluation and management service. If the admitting physician only reviews this information, he/she would "count" this under the medical decision making portion of his/her service. If, however, the admitting physician reviews the information with the patient and adds to the information, he/she may count this as actually taking a history, but only to the extent that he/she augments the existing history.

Coverage Issues

Carrier Bulletins

If the carrier published information about coverage of a particular service and the provider bills incorrectly, resulting in incorrect payment, is the physician liable?

Yes. The physician is responsible for billing in accordance with Medicare guidelines. Additionally, the physician would also be responsible for guidelines published in the AMA's CPT manual.

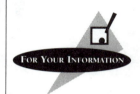

The physician is responsible for billing in accordance with Medicare guidelines.

Chiropractic Coverage

What are the requirements for Medicare coverage for chiropractic services?

The definition of a chiropractor, according to HCFA, is a physician that performs services for the purpose of manual manipulation of the spine to correct a subluxation demonstrated by x-ray. In accordance with the Balanced Budget Act of 1996, effective Jan. 1, 2000, the requirement of an x-ray demonstrating the presence of subluxation has been eliminated. Medicare Part B will now pay for a subluxation if the subluxation has resulted in a neuromusculoskeletal condition for which manipulation is the appropriate treatment, without the need of a x-ray.

Covered Visit with Preventive Care

If a Medicare patient was treated for an illness but also had a preventive physical on the same day, does Medicare cover any of the visit?

According to the Medicare Carriers Manual, when the physician furnishes a Medicare beneficiary a covered visit at the same place and on the same occasion as a preventive medicine service (CPT codes 99381-99397), the covered visit will be considered in lieu of a part of the preventive medicine service of equal value to the visit. A preventive medicine service (99381-99397) is a noncovered service for Medicare. The physician may charge the beneficiary for the noncovered remainder of the service, the amount by which the physician's current established charge for the preventive medicine service exceeds his/her current established charge for the covered visit. The physician is not required to give the beneficiary written advance notice of noncoverage for the part of the visit that constitutes a routine preventive visit. However, the physician is responsible for notifying the patient in advance of his/her liability for the charges for services that are not medically necessary to treat the illness or injury.

There could be covered and noncovered procedures performed during this encounter (e.g., screening x-ray, EKG, lab tests). These would be considered individually. Those procedures that are for screening for asymptomatic conditions are considered noncovered and, therefore, no payment would be made. Those procedures ordered to diagnose or monitor a symptom, medical condition, or treatment are evaluated for medical necessity and, if covered, are paid.

But because Medicare does not cover these services, they are not subject to the limiting charges. Claims for the covered portions of the service should be submitted along with noncovered portions of the service on the same claim form.

Physicians billing their claims electronically need to link the ICD-9-CM code with the appropriate procedure code. A nonparticipating physician who is not accepting assignment should use the limiting charge for 99213 instead of the allowable charges used by participating physicians, and follow the rest of the example above. For both participating and nonparticipating claims, services done routinely with the complete physical examination

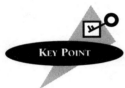

KEY POINT

Claims for the covered portions of the service should be submitted along with noncovered portions of the service on the same claim form.

that have not been linked to a covered medical diagnosis (for example, routine chest x-ray or routine EKG) would be denied and the patient will be responsible for those payments.

Diabetes Coverage

Are diabetes outpatient self-management training services covered by Medicare?

They are, under specified circumstances. Outpatient self-management training services may be covered under Medicare only if the physician who is managing the beneficiary's diabetic condition certifies that such services are needed under a comprehensive plan of care related to the beneficiary's diabetic condition to ensure therapy compliance or to provide the individual with necessary skills and knowledge in the management of the beneficiary's condition.

A certified provider (a physician or other individual or entity) provides other items and services for which payment may be made and meets certain quality standards. These certified providers must meet the National Diabetes Advisory Board Standards (NDAB). These services may be provided in two ways. First, the services performed by nonphysician providers may be incident-to a physician's professional services and must be performed under the physician's direct personal supervision. Secondly, a nonphysician practitioner, such as a physician assistant or nurse practitioner may be licensed under State law to perform a specific medical procedure and may be able to perform the procedure without physician supervision and have the services separately covered and paid for directly by Medicare as physician assistant or nurse practitioner services.

These services are coded with HCPCS Level II codes G0108 and G0109.

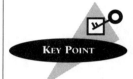

KEY POINT

Services performed by nonphysician providers may be incident-to a physician's professional services and must be performed under the physician's direct personal supervision.

Quick Guide to Physician Fraud and Abuse Prevention

Is a continuous subcutaneous insulin (CSII) pump covered by HCFA for patients who have a diagnosis of diabetes?

Yes. HCFA will cover the pump when it has been determined the device is medically necessary. Medical documentation must be submitted to ascertain medical necessity. The CSII pump and supplies should be billed using the following codes:

- E0784—External ambulatory infusion pump, insulin
- J1820—Injection, insulin, up to 100 units
- A4230, A4231, A4232—Supplies for insulin pump

The applicable ICD-9-CM diagnostic codes are:

250.01	250.03	250.11	250.13	250.21
250.23	250.31	250.33	250.41	250.43
250.51	250.53	250.61	250.63	250.71
250.73	250.81	250.83	250.91	250.93

Dietitians' Services

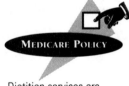

MEDICARE POLICY

Dietitian services are noncovered services under the Part B Medicare program when performed in a physician's office.

How can I bill for dietitian services provided in my office?

Dietitian services are noncovered services under the Part B Medicare program when performed in a physician's office because dietitians are not considered limited licensed practitioners and therefore the services they provide are not separately billable. However, if the dietitian's services are provided "incident to" a physician's professional services (e.g., the dietitian provides diabetic counseling to a patient the physician is treating for diabetes), the services would be covered under the "incident to" provision.

Locum Tenens

What is locum tenens?

Locum tenens is a long-standing and widespread practice whereby physicians retain substitute physicians to take over their professional practices when the regular physicians are absent for reasons such as illness, pregnancy, vacation, or continuing education. As part of this

Coverage Issues

arrangement, the regular physician bills and receives payment for the substitute physician's services as though he/she performed them himself/herself. The substitute physician generally has no practice of his/her own and moves from area to area as needed. The regular physician generally pays the substitute physician a fixed amount per diem, with the substitute physician having the status of an independent contractor rather than that of an employee. These substitute physicians are generally called "locum tenens" physicians.

What is covered under the locum tenens arrangement? Are there certain criteria that must be met for the regular physician to submit a claim?

A patient's regular physician may submit a claim for covered visit services (including emergency visits and related services) for a locum tenens physician who is not an employee of the regular physician and whose services are provided for patients of the regular physician's offices, if:

- The regular physician is unavailable to provide the visit services

- The Medicare beneficiary arranges or seeks to receive the visit services from the regular physician

- The regular physician pays the locum tenens physician for his/her services on a per diem or similar fee-for-time basis

- The substitute physician does not provide the visit services to Medicare patients over a continuous period of longer than 60 days

- The regular physician identifies the services as "substitute physician services" by appending HCPCS Level II modifier -Q6 (service rendered by a locum tenens physician) to the procedure code reported in Item 24d of the HCFA-1500 form. When the HCFA-1500 form is next revised, provisions will be made to identify the substitute physician by entering his/her

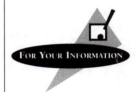

For Your Information

A patient's regular physician may submit a claim for covered visit services for a locum tenens physician.

97

Quick Guide to Physician Fraud and Abuse Prevention

unique physician identification number (UPIN) on the form and cross-referring the entry to the appropriate service line item (B) by number(s). HCFA has indicated that, until further notice, the regular physician must keep a record on file of each service provided by the substitute physician (associated with the substitute physician's UPIN), and make this record available to the Medicare carrier upon request

The requirements listed also apply when a medical group submits claims for services rendered by a locum tenens physician to patients of the regular physician, who is a member of that medical group. For purposes of these requirements, per diem or similar fee-for-time compensation that the group pays the locum tenens physician is considered paid by the regular physician. Also, a physician who left the group and for whom the group engaged a locum tenens physician as a temporary replacement may still be considered a member of the group until a permanent replacement is obtained. The group member must enter HCPCS Level II modifier -Q6 after the procedure code in Item 24d of the HCFA-1500 claim form and maintain a record of each service provided by the substitute physician associated with the substitutive physician's UPIN, and make this record available to the Medicare carrier upon request. Additionally, the medical group physician for whom the substitution services were rendered must be identified via his/her provider identification number in Item 24k of the appropriate line item of the HCFA-1500 claim form or electronic media equivalent.

Note: Postoperative services that a substitute physician renders during the period covered by the global fee do not need to be identified on the claim as substitution services.

Coverage Issues

Medical Necessity Denials

How can a physician, provider, or supplier who has accepted assignment and has no patient contact (such as a laboratory or radiologist) be expected to know whether a service will be denied as not medically necessary, and to furnish the beneficiary with a notice that the service will most likely be denied as not medically necessary?

Despite the fact that some physicians, providers, or suppliers may have limited contact with patients, they are expected to be aware of both national coverage policy and current local medical review policy. In the absence of a national coverage policy, local medical review policy indicates which items/services the Medicare carrier will cover, and under what clinical circumstances these items/services will be considered reasonable, medically necessary, and appropriate. In most cases, the availability of this information indicates that the physician, provider, or supplier knew, or should have known, that the item/service would be denied as not medically necessary. Furthermore, if there is a question regarding the number of times a service has been furnished to the beneficiary within a specific period, the physician, provider or supplier should clarify this information with either the beneficiary or the physician who ordered the tests.

If, after considering national coverage policy, local medical review policy, and any additional pertinent information, the physician, provider, or supplier believes there is a likelihood that the item/service may be denied as not medically necessary, the physician, provider, or supplier should furnish the beneficiary with proper advance notice to that effect. Such a notice serves as proof that the beneficiary had knowledge prior to the furnishing of the item/service that it would most likely be denied as not medically necessary. If no such notice was furnished, the physician, provider, or supplier could be held liable for the charge if it is determined that he/she knew, or should have known, that the item/service would be denied as not medically necessary.

In cases where a supplier is merely furnishing items/services (e.g., tests) ordered by another physician, if the ordering physician provides the beneficiary with proper advance notice that the ordered item/service may not be medically necessary, that notice would relieve the physician, provider, or supplier furnishing the item/service of liability for the charge. In this case, however, if the question of knowledge were to arise, the physician, provider, or supplier would have to submit to Medicare a copy of the written advance notice that was given to the beneficiary by the ordering physician or, if the written advance notice is determined to be unacceptable (e.g., it does not meet the advance notice language requirements), the provider or supplier will not be protected by that notice and can be held liable.

The protection against liability that may be provided to a furnishing provider or supplier by another entity's (namely the ordering physician's) advance notice to the beneficiary applies only in those situations where a provider or supplier is merely furnishing items/services ordered by that other entity. In cases where a physician makes a referral to another physician, provider, or supplier, any advance notice that is given to the beneficiary by the referring physician concerning the likelihood of denial on the basis of medical necessity cannot provide the entity to which the beneficiary is referred, with protection against liability for the items/services it furnishes the beneficiary. In such cases, the furnishing provider or supplier is in the best position to evaluate the likelihood of Medicare coverage or denial of the items/services and, therefore, is responsible for giving proper advance notice to the beneficiary. To be protected under the limitation of liability provision, the furnishing physician, provider, or supplier must give his/her own proper advance notice to the beneficiary for any items/services that he/she believes are likely to be denied as not medically necessary.

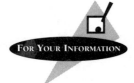

For Your Information

The furnishing provider or supplier is in the best position to evaluate the likelihood of Medicare coverage or denial of the items/services.

Coverage Issues

Noncovered Services and Supplies

How do we identify the services and supplies that are noncovered by Medicare?

The Medicare Carriers Manual states that no payment will be made for the following items and services:

- Services and items that are not reasonable and necessary
- Services or items for which there is no legal obligation to pay for or provide services (e.g., indigency, patient has other insurance, replacement of a warrantied item)
- Services or items furnished or paid for by government instrumentalities
- Services or items not provided within the United States
- Services resulting from war
- Personal comfort items or services
- Routine services and appliances
- Supportive devices for feet
- Custodial care
- Cosmetic surgery
- Charges for services/items provided to immediate relatives or members of household
- Dental services
- Services or items that are paid or expected to be paid under worker's compensation
- Nonphysician services provided to a hospital inpatient that were not provided directly or arranged for by the hospital

In addition, services related to noncovered services are also noncovered. Medical services required to treat a condition that arises as a result of a noncovered service — including services related to follow-up care and complications of noncovered services that require treatment during a

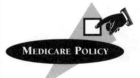

Services related to noncovered services are also noncovered.

Quick Guide to Physician Fraud and Abuse Prevention

hospital stay during which the noncovered service was performed — are not covered services under Medicare.

The following are examples of services "related to" and "not related to" noncovered services provided while the beneficiary was an inpatient:

- The patient was hospitalized for a noncovered service and broke a leg while in the hospital. Services related to care of the broken leg during this stay are "not related to" services and are covered under Medicare

- A patient was admitted to the hospital for covered services, but during the course of hospitalization became a candidate for a noncovered transplant or implant and actually received the transplant or implant during that hospital stay. When an original admission is entirely unrelated to the diagnosis that leads to a recommendation for a noncovered transplant or implant, the services related to the admitting condition would be covered

- After a patient has been discharged from a hospital stay during which he/she received noncovered services, medical and hospital services required to treat a condition or complication that arises as a result of the prior noncovered services may be covered when they are reasonable and necessary in all other respects. Thus, coverage could be provided for subsequent inpatient stays or outpatient treatment ordinarily covered by Medicare, even if the need for treatment arose because of a previous noncovered procedure. Some examples of services that may be found to be covered under this policy are the reversal of intestinal bypass surgery for obesity, repair of a noncovered bladder stimulator, or treatment of any infection at the surgical site of a noncovered transplant that occurred following discharge from the hospital. However, any subsequent services that could be expected to have been incorporated into a global fee should be denied. Thus, when a patient undergoes cosmetic surgery and the treatment regimen calls for a series of

Coverage Issues

postoperative visits to the surgeon for evaluating the patient's progress, these visits should be denied

Nonphysician Practitioners

Does Medicare allow payment for nurse practitioners, clinical nurse specialists, and physician assistants?

Yes, but only under specific guidelines. Payments to nurse practitioners and clinical nurse specialists have increased, as well as the removal of restrictions on settings for services furnished by nurse practitioners (NP) and clinical nurse specialists (CNS). They may be paid in all settings if no facility or other provider charges are paid in connection with the service. Payment would be equal to 80 percent of the lesser of the actual charge or 85 percent of the physician fee schedule. Payment could be made directly to the NP or CNS.

For physician assistants (PAs), restrictions that were previously put on settings and services furnished have been removed. Payments are allowed for services furnished by PAs in all settings but only if no facility or other provider charges is paid in connection with the service. Payment would equal 80 percent of the lesser of the actual charge or 85 percent of the physician fee schedule. Because PA payment is made only to the employer, payment is allowed to a PA as an independent contractor to qualify as an employment relationship.

Optometrist Services

Does Medicare cover optometrists' services?

Before 1987, the services of optometrist were covered only if related to the condition of aphakia. The Omnibus Budget Reconciliation Act of 1986, made an amendment expanding coverage for optometrist services. This amendment states that services are covered by Medicare if the optometrist is legally authorized to perform as a doctor of optometry by the State in which the optometrist performs them.

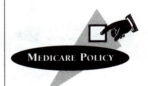
MEDICARE POLICY

Services are covered by Medicare if the optometrist is legally authorized to perform as a doctor of optometry by the State in which the optometrist performs them.

103

In the *Federal Register*, dated July 22, 1999, Volume 64, No. 140, conforms the regulations to be consistent with the statutory provision that has been implemented through manual provisions. The regulations specify that Medicare Part B pays for the services of a doctor of optometry, acting within the scope of his/her license, if the services would be covered as physicians' services when performed by a doctor of medicine or osteopathy.

I am an optometrist who has patients in nursing homes. Will Medicare cover my visits to these patients without their attending physicians having to write orders for my services?

Under the Social Security Act, the term, "physician" means a doctor of medicine or osteopathy, a doctor of dental surgery or of dental medicine, a doctor of podiatric medicine, a doctor of optometry, or a chiropractor. Therefore, if you have an ongoing physician-patient relationship with the resident of a nursing home, that person's attending physician does not have to write an order for your services. However, if you have not provided any professional services to this person for three years, this person would be considered a "new patient." In that situation, you would need an order for your services from this patient's attending physician.

Outside Lab Orders

Are physicians required to give the patient advance notice when ordering routine tests at an outside laboratory?

Physicians are not required to give patients advance notice for routine screening services that are not covered under Medicare Part B. However, many have found that advising the patient of noncoverage of routine services is good business practice.

MEDICARE POLICY

Physicians are not required to give patients advance notice for routine screening services that are not covered under Medicare Part B.

Coverage Issues

Pap Smears

Is a diagnostic pap smear covered under Medicare Part B?

A diagnostic pap smear and related medically necessary services are covered under Medicare Part B when ordered by a physician under one of the following conditions:

- Previous cancer of the cervix, uterus, or vagina that has been or is presently being treated

- Previous abnormal pap smear

- Any abnormal findings of the vagina, uterus, ovaries, or adnexa

- Any significant complaint by the patient referable to the female reproductive system

- Any signs or symptoms that might, in the physician's judgement, reasonably be related to a gynecological disorder

Physician Orders and Pneumococcal Pneumonia Vaccine (PPV)

Is a physician order (written or oral), plan of care, or any other type of physician involvement required for Medicare coverage of PPV?

Yes. Unless PPV is administered under the supervision of a physician, Medicare requires either a prescription written specifically for the beneficiary who is receiving PPV, or a previously written physician order (standing order). The standing order must specify that the individual or entity providing PPV must:

- Determine the person's age, health, and vaccination status

- Obtain a signed consent

- Administer an initial dose of PPV only to persons at high risk of pneumococcal disease

- Re-vaccinate only persons at highest risk of serious pneumococcal infection and those likely to have a

Quick Guide to Physician Fraud and Abuse Prevention

rapid decline in pneumococcal antibody levels, provided that at least five (5) years have passed since receipt of a previous dose of PPV

- Provide a record of vaccination to the patient

Physician Referral

What constitutes a physician referral?

A physician makes a referral when he/she makes a request for an item or service covered by Medicare Part B. It includes situations in which a physician requests a consultation (an opinion or advice) with another physician and covers any test or procedure that the other physician orders, performs, or supervises.

A physician also makes a referral for Part A or Part B services when he/she requests or establishes a plan of care that includes designated health services to be provided to a patient.

Pneumococcal Pneumonia Vaccine (PPV) and the Limiting Charge

Does the limiting charge provision apply to the PPV benefit?

No. Nonparticipating physicians and suppliers who do not accept assignment for the PPV benefit may collect their usual charges (i.e., the amount charged a patient who is not a Medicare beneficiary) for PPV and its administration. The beneficiary is responsible for paying the difference between what the physician or supplier charges and the amount Medicare allows.

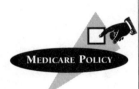

MEDICARE POLICY

PPV Benefit
The beneficiary is responsible for paying the difference between what the physician or supplier charges and the amount Medicare allows.

Podiatry in Nursing Homes

I am a podiatrist who has been rendering routine foot care to a nursing home resident who now needs a complete nail excision. Will I need an order for this surgery from the patient's attending physician in order for the surgery to be covered by Medicare?

Under the Social Security Act, the term, "physician" means a doctor of medicine or osteopathy, a doctor of dental surgery or of dental medicine, a doctor of podiatric medicine, a doctor of optometry, or a chiropractor. Therefore, if you have an ongoing physician-patient relationship with the resident of a nursing home, that person's attending physician does not have to write an order for your services. However, if you have not provided any professional services to this person for three years, this person would be considered a "new patient," and you would, in that situation, require an order for your services from this patient's attending physician.

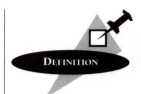

DEFINITION

Physician
A doctor of medicine or osteopathy, a doctor of dental surgery or of dental medicine, a doctor of podiatric medicine, a doctor of optometry, or a chiropractor.

PPV and Part A

Is a person with only Part A coverage entitled to receive PPV and have it covered under Part B?

No. PPV and its administration are a Part B covered service only.

RNs and PPV

May a registered nurse, employed by a physician, use the physician's provider number if the nurse, in a location other than the physician's office, provides a pneumococcal pneumonia vaccine (PPV)?

If the nurse is not working for the physician when the services are provided (e.g., a nurse is "moonlighting," administering PPV at a shopping mall at his or her own direction and not that of the physician), the nurse may obtain a provider number and bill the carrier directly. However, if the nurse is working for the physician when the services are provided, the nurse would use the physician's provider number for reporting purposes.

Second Opinions

Are second opinions considered referrals?

Second or third opinions are not considered to be referrals as long as they are initiated by the patient and are limited in nature — a one time service, for example.

Telephone Orders

Can an attending physician authorize an order for a service or procedure over the telephone?

Yes, provided the attending physician subsequently signs the order and documents the medical necessity of the service or procedure in the medical record.

Telephone Referrals

Can an attending physician authorize over the telephone the referral of a nursing facility resident to another provider specialty?

Yes, provided the physician subsequently signs the order for the referral and documents the medical necessity of the referral in the medical record.

Treating Relatives

Are services provided by a physician to his/her relatives covered by Medicare if they are Medicare beneficiaries?

Medicare does not pay for services usually covered under Medicare if the charges for those services are generated by an immediate relative of the physician or to a member of the physician's immediate household. This exclusion is intended to prevent Medicare payment for items and services provided by physicians and suppliers that would ordinarily be furnished gratuitously because of their relationship to the patient.

Coverage Issues

The Medicare Carriers Manual identifies the following degrees of relationship to be included within the definition of immediate relative:

- Husband or wife
- Natural or adoptive parent, child, or sibling
- Stepparent, stepchild, stepbrother, or stepsister
- Father-in-law, mother-in-law, son-in-law, daughter-in-law, brother-in-law, sister-in-law
- Grandparent or grandchild
- Spouse of grandparent or grandchild

Note: For Medicare's purposes, a brother-in-law or sister-in-law relationship is not considered to exist between a physician (or supplier) and the spouse of his wife's (her husband's) brother or sister. In addition, a father-in-law or mother-in-law relationship is not considered to exist between a physician and his/her spouse's stepfather or stepmother.

A member of the immediate household is defined as a person sharing a common abode with the patient as part of a single family unit and includes those individuals related by blood, marriage, or adoption, as well as domestic employees and others living together as part of a single family unit. Roomers and boarders are not included in this definition.

Quick Guide to Physician Fraud and Abuse Prevention

Vaccination Status for Pneumococcal Pneumonia Vaccine (PPV)

Does a beneficiary have to provide something in writing to show his/her vaccination status in order to obtain the pneumococcal pneumonia vaccine? Is it necessary for the provider to review the beneficiary's medical records?

No. Individuals and entities providing PPV to Medicare beneficiaries may rely on an oral account of vaccination status provided by a competent beneficiary.

Legislation/Legal Issues

A Definition of "Overpayment"

What is meant by an "overpayment"?

When a practice receives more reimbursement for a service than is allowed by Medicare, it has received an overpayment. If this happens, notify your carrier in writing. Be sure that you get written confirmation from the carrier that it has received the overpayment notification. Otherwise, there is no proof that the carrier received it, and such proof may be necessary later to show that the practice did not intentionally accept the overpayment.

Overpayments can occur for a variety of reasons, some of which are described below:

- Payment is made by both Medicare and another payer
- Payment is sent to the provider instead of the patient
- An error occurs in the calculation of the deductible or coinsurance
- A computer or clerical error is made (e.g., same charge processed twice)
- Payment is made for noncovered items and services, including those that are not medically necessary
- Payment is provided even though another payer is primary
- Payment is in excess of the Medicare allowed amount

Regardless of how an overpayment occurs, Medicare expects providers to correct the error and return the excess payment. This amount of money is a debt owed to the federal government and should not be taken lightly. If a

DEFINITION

Overpayment
When a practice receives more reimbursement for a service than is allowed by Medicare, it has received an overpayment

pattern of overpayments occurs, the practice could be investigated for fraud.

Anti-Kickback Statute and Referral Prohibitions

What is the difference between the Anti-Kickback Statute and the physician referral prohibitions in the Social Security Act?

The Anti-Kickback Statute is a criminal statute that applies to individuals or entities who knowingly and willfully offer, pay, solicit, or receive remuneration to induce the furnishing of items or services covered by Medicare or state health care programs (including Medicaid), or any state programs receiving funds under titles V or XX of the Social Security Act. In the original Anti-Kickback Statute, offenses that were classified as felonies were punishable by fines of up to $25,000 or imprisonment for up to five years, or both. The Balanced Budget Act (BBA) of 1997 increased civil fines to $50,000 for each violation of the Anti-Kickback Statute, added a provision for damages up to three times the amount of the illegal kickback paid, and added monetary penalties for individuals who knowingly contract with sanctioned persons or entities. In addition, entities and individuals that violate the Anti-Kickback Statute can be excluded from Medicare and state health care programs.

The safe harbor regulations identify practices that are protected from criminal prosecution or civil sanctions under the Anti-Kickback Statute.

The physician self-referral law, also referred to as Stark I and II, prohibits physicians from referring Medicare patients to certain entities for designated health services if the physician (or an immediate family member) has a financial relationship with the entity. The law also prohibits Medicare payments for any designated health service provided in violation of the law. If a person collects any amount for services billed in violation of the law, he/she must make a refund. A person can be subject to a civil money penalty or exclusion from Medicare, Medicaid, and

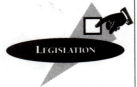

LEGISLATION

The law also prohibits Medicare payments for any designated health service provided in violation of the law.

other programs if that person (1) presents or causes to be presented a claim to Medicare or a bill to any individual, third-party payer, or other entity for any designated health service the person knows or should know was furnished as the result of a prohibited referral, or (2) fails to make a timely refund.

Attorney-Client Privilege

What's "attorney-client privilege"?

The attorney-client privilege is a principle or doctrine that excludes from discovery or evidences nearly all written and oral communications between an attorney and his/her client. This privilege could be one of the most important protections available to your practice. You may discover problems during your compliance audit that requires the immediate attention of an attorney. When the attorney-client privilege is in place, no one can be compelled to testify about the discussions between the lawyer and the client, even when past or potential violations of the law were discussed.

There is only one major exception to this privilege; as one court put it, "a quid pro quo is exacted for the attorney-client confidence: the client must not abuse the confidential relation by using it to further a fraudulent or criminal scheme."

DEFINITION

Attorney-Client Privilege
The attorney-client privilege is a principle or doctrine that excludes from discovery or evidences nearly all written and oral communications between an attorney and his/her client.

Attorney's Role in Compliance

How should our attorney function in our compliance plan?

The role of legal counsel in the compliance plan may differ based on the size of the practice. A solo practitioner will have different needs than a large multi-specialty practice based on, for example, the average number of claims, the number of personnel the practice employs, variable procedures and services, and, more than likely, business arrangements and sites of services. Some practices choose

Quick Guide to Physician Fraud and Abuse Prevention

to appoint their legal counsel as the compliance officer or a member of their compliance committee.

No matter how complex the compliance plan, the attorney's most important responsibilities are to (1) provide legal advice, within the context of the compliance plan, about how to take legal actions to avoid being investigated or being prosecuted, and (2) defend the practice when it is being investigated or being prosecuted. With this in mind, if you suspect that actions occurred that might lead to criminal or civil liability for an individual employee or the practice as a whole, your attorney should be notified immediately so that he/she can advise you of the appropriate actions to be taken, and possibly to perform or coordinate an internal investigation.

The attorney's initial involvement in the compliance plan should be limited to conducting a preliminary overview to identify problem areas, possible causes, and obvious investigative targets. The attorney also should make himself/herself familiar with the practice's organizational structure, business arrangements, and billing procedure requirements that the practice's personnel are required to follow.

The responsibility for legal decisions (e.g., whether to disclose facts or terminate an employee, or how to correct identified problems) ultimately rests with legal counsel, the physician(s), and the practice administrator/manager.

Beneficiaries and Fraud and Abuse

How are beneficiaries involved in the fight against fraud and abuse?

Anti-Fraud messages are located in the Medicare Handbook, which is the information that is given to all beneficiaries. This states that the Handbook must contain four elements:

- A statement indicating that errors occur and Medicare fraud, waste, and abuse is a significant problem and

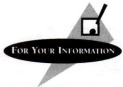

For Your Information

The responsibility for legal decisions ultimately rests with legal counsel, the physician(s), and the practice administrator/manager.

Legislation/Legal Issues

encourage beneficiaries to review any Explanation of Medicare Benefits for accuracy and to report errors or questionable charges

- A description of a beneficiary's right to request an itemized statement from their provider for Medicare items and services

- A description of the beneficiary incentive program established under HIPAA

- The Health and Human Services Inspector Generals toll-free hotline number, which receives complaints and information about waste, fraud, and abuse

In addition to the four elements, the Explanation of Medicare Benefits (EOMB) are required to contain a list of items and/or services provided to the beneficiary and the amount of payment for each item and/or services. The beneficiary has the opportunity to request an itemized statement from the provider in writing, if they wish to do so. The written request is made to the physician for the itemized statement, and if the statement is not furnished within 30 day of such a notice, a Civil Monetary Penalty may be imposed. The beneficiary may submit this to the appropriate governmental entity for review and they will determine the accuracy of the statement and recover any erroneous payments, if applicable. The EOMB is being replaced with a Medicare Summary Notice (MSN), which will provide the beneficiary with a monthly summary of all Medicare claims filed as well as periodic messages pertinent to the beneficiary such as the fraud and abuse hotline number. MSNs are being phased in over several years, but are already being used by some Medicare contractors.

Civil Investigative Demand

What is a "civil investigative demand"?

A civil investigative demand is the issuance (by the Justice Department over the signature of the Attorney General) of a subpoena for investigating issues of fraud and abuse in the form of interrogatories. In other words, a civil

115

Quick Guide to Physician Fraud and Abuse Prevention

investigative demand authorizes the Justice Department to set in motion a process by which a set of formal questions can be asked in order that pertinent information can be exchanged between the defendant's and the plaintiff's counsels in the discovery phase of a legal suit.

The 1996 Health Insurance Portability and Accountability Act (HIPAA) provisions also created additional "authorized investigative demand" procedures, pursuant to which the Attorney General issues subpoenas in health care fraud cases. These provisions require:

- The production of any records that may be relevant to an authorized law enforcement inquiry, that a person or entity may possess
- A custodian of records to give testimony concerning the production and authentication of such records

Civil Monetary Penalties

What are Civil Monetary Penalties (CMPs)?

In 1981, Congress added section 1128A to the Social Security Act to authorize the Secretary of Health and Human Services the ability to impose civil monetary penalties. These civil monetary penalties are financial penalties due to the damages the governmental agency has sustained because of a health care claim that had been filed. Since 1981, Congress has increased the number and types of circumstances under which CMPs may be imposed. Statutory provisions are also in place, which allow the Secretary to impose additional monetary payments for statutory violations. The original penalty was $2,000 per item or service and twice the amount claimed. The Health Insurance Portability and Accountability Act of 1996 provided a law for a higher penalty ($10,000 per item or service) and a higher assessment, to three times the amount claimed.

Any individual excluded from Medicare or a state health program who retains either direct or indirect ownership or control in an entity participating in Medicare, and any

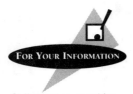

For Your Information

Civil monetary penalties are financial penalties due to the damages the governmental agency has sustained because of a health care claim that had been filed.

116

Legislation/Legal Issues

individual who knows or should have known the basis for an exclusion, or who is an officer or managing employee of the entity, is subject to a civil monetary penalty of not more than $10,000 for each day the relationship continues.

Civil monetary penalties of not more than three times the amount of the payments or $5,000, whichever is greater, will be imposed on physicians who falsely certify that a patient meets Medicare's requirements for home health care.

Additional practices that are subject to civil monetary penalties are improper coding and attempts to obtain reimbursement for services that are not medically necessary. Penalties of up to $10,000 may be imposed for each instance of medically unnecessary services.

According to the Social Security Act, a Civil Monetary Penalty of up to $50,000 plus up to three times the amount of the remuneration offered, paid solicited, or received could be levied for each violation of the Anti-Kickback provisions.

Under what circumstances may HCFA apply civil monetary penalties, assessments, and/or exclusions?

Civil monetary penalties, assessments, and/or exclusions may be imposed by HCFA for program noncompliance under the following circumstances:

1. Any person billing for a clinical diagnostic laboratory test, other than on an assignment-related basis. This provision includes tests performed in a physician's office but excludes tests performed in a rural health clinic. (This violation is subject to a CMP, assessment, and exclusion.)

2. Any person billing for an intraocular lens inserted during or after cataract surgery for which payment may be made for services in an ambulatory surgical center. (This violation is subject to a CMP.)

Quick Guide to Physician Fraud and Abuse Prevention

3. When seeking payment on an unassigned basis, any entity failing to provide information about a referring physician, including the referring physician's name and unique physician identification number. (This violation is subject to a CMP and exclusion.)

4. Any nonparticipating physician charging a Medicare beneficiary more than the limiting charge for radiologist services. (This violation is subject to a CMP, assessment, and exclusion.)

5. Any nonparticipating physician charging a Medicare beneficiary more than the limiting charge for mammography screening. (This violation is subject to a CMP, assessment, and exclusion.)

6. For health care practitioners (physician assistants, nurse practitioners, clinical nurse specialists, certified registered nurse anesthetists, certified nurse-midwives, clinical social workers, and clinical psychologists), any health care practitioner billing (or collecting) for any services on a nonassigned basis. (This violation is subject to a CMP, assessment, and exclusion.)

7. Any physician presenting a claim or bill for an assistant at cataract surgery performed on or after March 1, 1987. (This violation is subject to a CMP, assessment, and exclusion.)

8. Any nonparticipating physician who does not accept payment on an assigned basis and who fails to refund beneficiaries for services that are not reasonable or medically necessary or are of poor quality. (This violation is subject to a CMP, assessment, and exclusion.)

9. Any nonparticipating physician billing for an elective surgical procedure on a nonassigned basis and whose charge is at least $500 and fails to disclose charge and coinsurance amounts to the Medicare beneficiary prior to rendering the service; and fails to refund any amount collected for the procedure in excess of the charges

118

Legislation/Legal Issues

recognized and approved by the Medicare program. (This violation is subject to a CMP, assessment, and exclusion.)

10. Any physician billing diagnostic tests in excess of the scheduled fee amount. (This violation is subject to a CMP, assessment, and exclusion.)

11. Any physician failing to promptly provide the appropriate diagnosis code or codes upon request by HCFA or a carrier on any request for payment or bill submitted on a nonassigned basis. (This violation is subject to a CMP.)

12. Any physician failing to provide the diagnosis code or codes after repeatedly being notified by HCFA of the obligations on any request for payment of bill submitted on a nonassigned basis. (This violation is subject to an exclusion.)

13. Any nonparticipating physician or other person who furnishes physicians' services and bills on a nonassigned basis or collects in excess of the limiting charge; or fails to make an adjustment or refund to the Medicare beneficiary. (This violation is subject to a CMP, assessment, and exclusion.)

14. Any person billing for physicians' services on a nonassigned basis for a Medicare beneficiary who is also eligible for Medicaid (these individuals include qualified Medicare beneficiaries). This provision applies to services furnished on or after April 1, 1990. (This violation is subject to a CMP, assessment, and exclusion.)

15. Any physician or other person (except those who have been excluded from the Medicare program) failing to submit a claim for a beneficiary within one year of providing the service; or imposes a charge for completing and submitting the standard claims form. (This violation is subject to a CMP and exclusion.)

Quick Guide to Physician Fraud and Abuse Prevention

Note: This list applies mainly to physicians. There are other civil monetary penalties, assessments, and exclusion that affect other health care entities.

Collections and the Limiting Charge

Can a physician sue patients in state small claims court to enforce collection of charges in excess of the limiting charge?

The practice of physicians suing patients in small claims court to recover excess payments above the Medicare limiting charge rates may very well violate federal law. If the charges in question constitute knowing, willful, and repeated violations of the charge limits, the Medicare program can impose sanctions. Also, in theory, the decisions of the small claims court could be set aside by the federal courts as inconsistent with Medicare law.

Consultants' Advice

If a consultant advises a physician to take certain actions that ultimately result in Medicare abuse or fraud, is the consultant then liable?

Because the decision to act was made by the physician, even though it was under incorrect advisement, the physician would in some circumstances be considered fully responsible.

Diagnostic Tests and Medical Necessity

When diagnostic tests are ordered and performed, who is responsible for ensuring that they were medically necessary?

It is the responsibility of a provider of the test to establish and document its medical necessity and to keep this on record for audit or review. There has been some confusion in this matter among providers, particularly providers of laboratory procedures or physiologic tests. If a provider or the testing facility is audited, there must be documentation

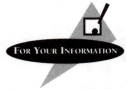

For Your Information

It is the responsibility of a provider of the test to establish and document its medical necessity and to keep this on record for audit or review.

Legislation/Legal Issues

on hand to substantiate the medical necessity of the procedure.

HCFA reimburses the testing facility or the provider of the service. Therefore, in a postpayment audit, this is where the recoupment will be made. In a postpayment audit, medical necessity must be established by adherence to nationally accepted standards of care and to Medicare guidelines. If Medicare reimburses you, you are responsible for establishing medical necessity.

A good example of this is a vascular laboratory to which a referring physician has sent a patient with a diagnosis of leg pain for an arterial study. The diagnosis of leg pain does not effectively justify the medical necessity of performing the test. There was no indication of ischemia, rest pain, or claudication involved in the diagnosis of leg pain. The diagnosis must be specific.

If this case were audited, Medicare would recoup any payment made for the test from the testing facility rather than the referring physician.

If the testing facility realizes that a diagnosis does not clearly indicate the medical necessity of an ordered test, the patient should be returned to the referring physician for substantiation of additional history before the test is performed. It would be in the best interest of the testing facility to establish internal guidelines and notify their referring physicians of these guidelines, making sure they do not conflict with national standards or Medicare guidelines, in order to ensure an audit trail of medical necessity.

> Note: The referring physician would be subject to civil monetary penalties for abusive practices if the ordering of tests that were not medically necessary (based on the diagnosis code reported) was found to be common in his/her practice pattern.

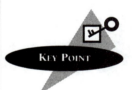

KEY POINT

The referring physician would be subject to civil monetary penalties for abusive practices if the ordering of tests that were not medically necessary was found to be common in his/her practice pattern.

121

Exclusion from Federal Health Care Programs

What types of items or services, when provided by excluded parties, violate an OIG exclusion?

If an excluded party supplies items or services, their employer or contractor may be liable for possible civil monetary penalties. This includes:

- Services performed by excluded nurses, technicians, or other excluded individuals who work for a hospital, nursing home, home health agency, or physician practice, where such services are related to administrative duties, preparation of surgical trays, or review of treatment plans if such services are reimbursed directly or indirectly (through a prospective payment or a bundled payment) by a federal health care program, even if the individuals do not furnish direct care to federal program beneficiaries

- Services performed by excluded pharmacists or other excluded individuals who input prescription information for pharmacy billing or who are involved in any way in filling prescriptions for drugs reimbursed, directly or indirectly, by any federal health care program

- Services performed by excluded ambulance drivers, dispatchers, and other employees involved in providing transportation reimbursed by a federal health care program, to hospital patients or nursing home residents

- Services performed by excluded social workers who are employed by health care entities to provide services to federal program beneficiaries, and whose services are reimbursed, directly or indirectly, by a federal health care program

- Services performed for program beneficiaries by excluded individuals who sell, deliver, or refill orders for medical devices or equipment being reimbursed by a federal health care program

Legislation/Legal Issues

- Administrative services, including the processing of claims for payment, performed for a Medicare intermediary or carrier, of a Medicaid fiscal agent, by an excluded individual
- Services performed by an excluded administrator, billing agent, accountant, claims processor, or utilization reviewer that are related to and reimbursed, directly or in indirectly, by a federal health care program
- Items of services provided to a program beneficiary by an excluded individual who works for an entity that has a contractual agreement with, and is paid by, a federal health care program
- Items of equipment sold by an excluded manufacturer or supplier, used in the care or treatment of beneficiaries and reimbursed, directly or indirectly, by a federal health care program

How do I know if an individual is excluded from a federally funded program?

There is a web site that has a list called, " OIG List of Excluded Individuals/Entities" on the OIG web site. This helps to avoid civil monetary penalty (CMP) liability. In addition to checking the web site, your health care provider should periodically check the OIG web site for determining the participation/exclusion status of current employees and contractors. The web site contains OIG program exclusion information and is updated in both on-line searchable and downloadable formats. This information is updated on a regular basis. The OIG web site sorts the exclusion of individuals and entities by: (1) the legal basis for the exclusion (2) the types of individuals and entities that have been excluded, and (3) the State where the excluded individual resided at the time they were excluded or the State where the entity was doing business.

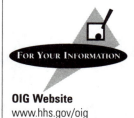

For Your Information

OIG Website
www.hhs.gov/oig

False Claims

What are the False Claims and Statement Acts?

There are three in place: The Criminal False Claims Act, Criminal False Statement Act, and the Civil False Claims Act, which are federal reimbursement statutes.

Criminal False Claims Act — This Act states that any provider who knowingly and willingly submits a false claim to the government may be found guilty of violating this Act. Penalties include fines of up to $10,000 and/or imprisonment for violations. The actual sentence will be driven by the Federal Sentencing Guidelines.

Criminal False Statements Act — This Act states that any provider who knowingly and willingly conceals or falsifies material facts, makes false statements, or submits false information of governmental documents, may be prosecuted under the Criminal False Statements Act. If found guilty, there is up to a $10,000 fine and/or imprisonment for up to five years.

Civil False Claims Act — Under the Civil False Claims Act, the provider may face civil prosecution for billing:

- Services or items the provider knows were not actually provided
- An incorrect code the provider knows will reimburse at a higher rate
- False codes
- Services as performed by a licensed professional when the services were actually performed by an unlicensed professional
- Services or items by individuals that have been sanctioned or excluded from governmental programs
- Services and procedures that the provider knows were not medically necessary

When violating any of these Acts, a provider may incur penalties that include fines of up to $10,000 for each false

Legislation/Legal Issues

claim, treble damages, and possible suspension and/or exclusion from federally funded health care programs. A provider who submits false claims to a federally funded program may be prosecuted under one or all or these Acts.

Fraud and Abuse Differentiated

What is the difference between fraud and abuse?

Medicare defines fraud as an intentional deception or misrepresentation that the individual knows to be false (or does not believe to be true) and knows could result in some unauthorized benefit to himself/herself or some other person.

Medicare defines abuse as incidents or practices that are inconsistent with accepted sound medical, business, or fiscal practices. These practices may directly or indirectly result in unnecessary costs to the program, improper payment, or payments for services that fail to meet professional recognized standards of care or that are medically unnecessary.

Note that the difference in the definitions of these two terms lies in the word "intentional." Also keep in mind that abusive situations may turn into fraudulent situations when a provider has been advised that certain practices are unacceptable, yet continues to follow the same abusive pattern.

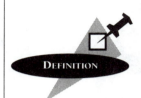

DEFINITION

Fraud
An intentional deception or misrepresentation that the individual knows to be false and knows could result in some unauthorized benefit to himself/herself or some other person.

Abuse
Incidents or practices that are inconsistent with accepted sound medical, business, or fiscal practices.

Fraud and Abuse Organizations

What organizations are involved in the fight against fraud and abuse?

All parties that deal with federal insurance programs would be included in the prevention and detection of fraud, waste, and abuse. This comprises such entities as the beneficiaries, Medicare contractors, providers, Peer Group Organizations (PGOs), State Medicaid Fraud Control Units (MFCUs), and federal agencies such as Health Care Financing Administration (HCFA), Office of the Inspector General

(OIG), Office of Investigations (OI) Field Office, Office of Audit Services (OAS), Federal Bureau of Investigation (FBI), Department of Justice (DOJ), and the Office of Civil Fraud and Administrative Adjudication (OCFAA). All of these organizations work together to ensure that only appropriate payments are made and all steps are taken to recover any overpayments that have been made to providers. They also are responsible to investigate and prosecute any party that has violated regulations and/or one who has committed fraud against federal insurance programs. Some of these Offices were created or expanded by the Health Insurance Portability and Accountability Act of 1996. This Act created a stable source for funding for program integrity activities (i.e., the development and/or expansion of some of the above Offices). In fiscal year 1999, $560 million was allocated; for fiscal year 2000, $630 million has been allocated.

Fraud by a Billing Company

Let's say a billing company is set up as the payee of a physician (on Medicare's file) and commits fraud by billing for additional services not rendered, does the physician have any responsibility for this situation?

Assuming the physician is not found responsible for any intentional wrongdoing by the court, the physician would not likely face prosecution. However, the physician would be responsible for refunding any overpaid monies to the Medicare program. This is because the physician, in entering into such an agreement with the billing company, extended authority for claim filing to the billing company. To prevent these types of situations from arising, the physician should have a process in place to periodically check his/her billed charges with those processed by Medicare to be sure they balance.

Legislation/Legal Issues

Healthcare Integrity and Protection Data Bank

I have heard of the Healthcare Integrity and Protection Data Bank (HIPDB), which used to be referred to as the Health Care Fraud and Abuse Data Collection Program. What is this program's purpose?

The purpose of the HIPDB program is to assure dissemination of information to governmental agencies and health care agencies regarding reportable offenses by providers, thereby preventing these providers from relocating and participating in Medicare or other federal health care programs in new locations. Federal and state agencies responsible for monitoring health care programs, and for some offenses, private health plans as well, must report a variety of final adverse actions including:

- Suspension or revocation of a state or federal license

- Reprimand or probation imposed by a state or federal licensing authority

- Voluntary surrender of a state or federal license

- Other "negative action" that is public information (e.g., imposition of fines for licensure violations)

- Criminal convictions related to the delivery of health care items or services

- Civil judgments related to the delivery of health care items or services

- Exclusion from participation in a federal or state health care program

A report must be made even if the result is a settlement or if the case is under appeal. Substantial penalties, $25,000 for each failure, may be levied against health plans for failure to report required information. However, there are a few penalties for reporting inaccurate information. Providers may challenge it within a fairly short time frame. Therefore, providers must monitor information in the data bank on a regular basis to assure that no incorrect information has been submitted.

127

Quick Guide to Physician Fraud and Abuse Prevention

Hospital Referrals and the Law

Why is it illegal for hospitals to provide financial incentives to physicians for their referrals?

These financial incentives violate the Anti-Kickback Statute. The OIG finds that these incentives interfere with a physician's duty to render the best care for his/her patients and can inflate Medicare costs by overusing the services of a particular hospital when treatment at that hospital may not be in the patient's best interest.

The OIG looks for the following in determining whether fraud exists:

- Payment of any sort of incentive by the hospital each time a physician refers a patient
- Provision of free or discounted office space or equipment
- Free or discounted billing, nursing, or staff services
- Free training for a physician's office staff in areas such as management techniques, CPT coding, and laboratory techniques
- Guarantees that provide that if the physician's income fails to reach a predetermined level, the hospital will supplement the income up to a certain amount
- Payment for physician continuing education courses
- The provision of low-interest or interest-free loans, or loans that may be "forgiven" if a physician refers patients to the hospital
- Payment of the cost of a physician's travel and expenses for conferences
- Insurance coverage provided under the hospital group health plan at a low cost
- Payment for services that require little, if any, substantive work by the physicians
- Payment for services to the physician that are in excess of fair market value

Legislation/Legal Issues

Improper Physician Certifications of Medical Necessity

What are the consequences when a physician signs a certification of medical necessity that may have false or misleading information?

If a physician knows the information is false, or acts with reckless disregard as to the truth of the statement, the physician risks criminal, civil, and administrative penalties. These include:

- Criminal prosecution
- Fines as high as $10,000 per false claim plus treble damages
- Administrative sanctions including exclusion from participation in federal health care programs, withholding or recovery of payments, and loss of license or disciplinary actions by state regulatory agencies

Inappropriate Certifications of Medical Necessity

What are some of the types of inappropriate certifications of medical necessity that are signed?

The OIG has uncovered numerous types of inappropriate certifications in the course of its investigations of fraud in the provision of home health services and medical equipment and supplies. These are:

- A signed certification as a "courtesy" to a patient, service, provider, or DME supplier when they have not first made a determination of medical necessity
- Knowingly or recklessly signing a false or misleading certification that causes a false claim to be submitted to a federal health care program
- Receiving any financial benefit for signing the certification (including free or reduced rent, patient referrals, supplies, equipment, or free labor)

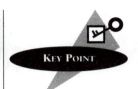

KEY POINT

If a physician knows the information is false, or acts with reckless disregard as to the truth of the statement, the physician risks criminal, civil, and administrative penalties.

129

Note: Even if the physician does not receive any financial gain or other benefit from providers or suppliers, they may be liable for making false statements or misleading certifications.

Examples of false or misleading certifications:

- Knowingly signing a number of forms provided by a home health agency that falsely represent that skilled nursing services are medically necessary in order to qualify that patient for home health services

- Certification of a patient to the home and that qualifies that patient for home health services although the patient tells the physician that her only restrictions are due to arthritis in her hands, and she has no restrictions on her routine activities, such as grocery shopping

- A stack of blank certification of medical necessity (CMNs) is signed for transcutaneous electrical stimulators (TENS) units. The CMNs are later completed with false information in support of fraudulent claims for the equipment. The false information shows that the physician ordered and certified the medical necessity for the TENS units for which the supplier has submitted claims

- CMNs are signed for wheelchairs and hospital beds without seeing the patients, then information is falsified in the medical charts to indicate that the physician has treated the patient

- A physician accepts a monetary gain from a durable medical supplier for each prescription that is signed for oxygen concentrators and nebulizers

Investment Interests

Is my membership in a nonprofit organization considered an investment interest and in violation of Stark regulations?

Not unless you or a family member receives compensation from the nonprofit organization.

Legislation/Legal Issues

Laundering of Monetary Instruments

What is laundering of monetary instruments?

Money laundering occurs when funds obtained illegally are mixed with funds obtained legally. Typically, the health care provider deposits all payments into a general account, whether they are payments from patients, Medicare, Medicaid, or other third party payers. Any deposit into a general account found to be the result of a fraudulent claim along with funds obtained by a legitimate claim may be interpreted as money laundering. A conviction on a health fraud offense can easily lead to an associated money laundering conviction.

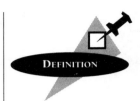

DEFINITION

Money laundering occurs when funds obtained illegally are mixed with funds obtained legally.

Limiting Charge Compliance Program

What is the Limiting Charge Compliance Program?

Congress enacted legislation in 1989 that established limits on nonparticipating physician charges. These "limiting charges" serve to protect Medicare beneficiaries from undue balance billing expenses. The limiting charge is 115 percent of the Medicare physician fee schedule and is applied to nonassigned claims.

Monitoring for limiting charge compliance is performed semi-monthly by the carrier. Limiting charge exception reports (LCERs) are sent to each physician if the carrier's records indicate the limiting charge has been exceeded on nonassigned claims processed during the preceding two weeks. Effective immediately, a tolerance of $1 will be applied to the monitoring process. This means that any charge that exceeds the limiting charge by more than $1 will cause an LCER to be produced. Previously, the tolerance was $5.

Please note that when a claim is reprocessed based on review and adjustment, it may appear on the LCER as a correction to the original claim if the original claim was deemed to be over the limiting charge. Amounts less than

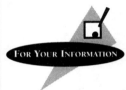

FOR YOUR INFORMATION

"Limiting charges" serve to protect Medicare beneficiaries from undue balance billing expenses.

131

$1 may appear based on review and adjustment of the original determination. In adjustment cases of less than $1, refunds to beneficiaries are not expected.

Medical Necessity Liability

If a physician refers a patient to another provider for diagnostic tests and the other provider bills medically unnecessary services as covered services, to what extent, if any, is the referring physician liable?

As long as the referral information concerning the diagnostic tests specifically documents the tests to be performed and the medical necessity of those tests as established by the diagnosis code(s), the referring physician would not be liable for any additional unnecessary services provided by the supplier of the tests. However, in the event that an investigation is pursued with the supplier regarding these additional unnecessary tests, the physician's records may be requested.

Most Favored Nation Clauses

What is the Most Favored Nation Clauses?

The most favored nation clauses typically require the provider to bill the third party payer the lowest fee charged to any other person or entity. Because HIPAA applies not only to Medicare and Medicaid, but to private health care plans as well, providers should review all third party contracts to verify that they are not required to waive copayments and deductibles.

Observation Care

Observation codes are confusing. What criteria are warranted for an admission to observation status?

The Medicare Carriers Manual specifically indicates that in order for a physician to bill the initial observation care codes, there must be a medical observation record for the patient that contains the physician's dated and timed admitting orders regarding the care the patient is to receive while in observation, nursing notes, and progress notes prepared by the physician while the patient was in observation status. This record must be in addition to any record prepared as a result of an emergency department or outpatient clinic encounter.

Professional Courtesy Discounts

We have given professional courtesy discounts in the past. Is this in violation of any federal health care regulation?

Providers may be in violation of federal and state anti-kickback laws if they submit claims to the patient's third party payer for the entire amount of the bill knowing at the time the claim was made that they would waive the copayment. The OIG has made it clear that routinely submitting claims for $100 for a third party payer when the provider is willing to accept $80 as payment in full may constitute a false entry. Routinely writing off copayments greatly increases the provider's chance of being successfully prosecuted.

Qui Tam

What is meant by "qui tam"?

The term "qui tam" is an abbreviation from the Latin "qui tam pro domino rege quam pro sic ipso in hoc parte sequitur," which means, "who as well for the king as for himself sues in this matter."

Qui tam is a provision of the Federal Civil False Claims Act that allows private citizens to file a lawsuit in the name of the US government charging fraudulent procurement of government funds, and share in any money recovered.

This unique law was enacted by Congress in order to effectively identify and prosecute government procurement and program fraud and recover revenue lost as a result of the fraud. The Qui tam provision has had the effect of

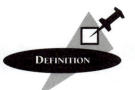

DEFINITION

Qui Tam
A provision of the Federal Civil False Claims Act that allows private citizens to file a lawsuit in the name of the US government charging fraudulent procurement of government funds, and share in any money recovered.

133

privatizing government legal remedies by allowing private citizens to act as "private attorney general" in the effort to prosecute illegal government procurement and program fraud.

Reacting to a Search Warrant

What should we do if we are confronted with a search warrant?

The best advice is to be prepared prior to the search. Designate a responsible individual as the investigation coordinator (or a team of coordinators if warranted by the size of the practice) to contact legal counsel upon receiving the warrant and to monitor the search.

The following procedures should be carried out or followed during the search:

- Identify and determine the affiliation of each of the investigators and which of these individuals is in charge
- Monitor only. Do not interfere as this can be misconstrued as obstruction of justice
- Take extensive notes regarding the questions asked, areas searched, and the records, hard drives, and documents seized
- If possible, get a copy of the affidavit in support of the warrant. In many cases this may be unavailable under seal. Immediately fax a copy to your attorney
- Request that all inquiries be directed to the investigation coordinator(s)
- Review the warrant. If the investigator is inspecting areas not specifically set forth in the warrant bring this to the investigator's attention. Be diplomatic as this also could be construed as obstruction of justice
- Request copies of the records, documents, files, and hard drives seized
- Identify attorney/client-privileged materials

Legislation/Legal Issues

As a part of your compliance plan you should establish written policies and procedures for your staff as to how to handle a search warrant or investigation notification.

Record Retention

How long should I keep my office medical records?

Each state has imposed its own specific record retention requirements for medical records in the statutes and regulations governing qualification for licensure. Because state laws are changing so quickly in this area, we can only recommend that you verify your state statutory and regulatory requirements. It is also advisable to verify retention requirements with your malpractice insurer.

Sanctions

What are the sanctions for individuals who have been convicted of a health crime?

According to Subtitle D, Anti-Fraud and Abuse Provisions, any individual who has been convicted on one previous occasion of one or more health-related crimes for which a mandatory exclusion could be imposed, including Medicare and State health care program-related crimes or felonies related to health care fraud, will be excluded from Medicare or any State health care program for at least 10 years. Any individual who has been convicted on two or more previous occasions of health care related crimes will be permanently excluded.

Also, if a person who, in anticipation of or following a conviction, assessment, or exclusion, transfers ownership or control of a health care entity to an immediate family member or member of the household, that health care entity will be excluded from Medicare or any State health care program.

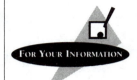

For Your Information

Each state has imposed its own specific record retention requirements for medical records in the statutes and regulations governing qualification for licensure.

135

"Standing Order" Defined

What is a standing order?

A standing order is a prescription written in advance by a responsible, identifiable physician to cover certain common treatment situations.

Waiving the Deductible and Copayment

Can I waive a patient's deductible and copayment?

The routine waiver of deductibles and copayments is unlawful because it results in false claims, violates the Anti-Kickback Statute, and constitutes excessive utilization of items and services paid by Medicare.

The provider or supplier who routinely waives Medicare deductibles and copayments is misrepresenting the actual charge of that service or supply. For instance, if the provider claims that the charge for a specific service is $100, but routinely waives the copayment, the actual charge is really $80. Medicare should be paying 80 percent of $80, which is $64, rather than 80 percent of $100, which is $80. Each time this service is billed, and the copayment waived, Medicare is paying $16 more for the service than it should be.

The exceptions to annual deductible and copayments are as follows:

- Pneumococcal vaccine and its administration
- Influenza virus vaccine and its administration
- Clinical diagnostic laboratory tests (including specimen collection fees) that are paid on an assigned basis or billed under the indirect payment procedure
- Part B home health services

Effective Jan. 1, 1998, the Balanced Budget Act of 1997 provided for the waiver of the deductible for screening mammographies and pelvic examinations.

MEDICARE POLICY

The routine waiver of deductibles and copayments is unlawful because it results in false claims, violates the Anti-Kickback Statute, and constitutes excessive utilization of items and services paid by Medicare.

Legislation/Legal Issues

When an Employee Commits Fraud

If an employee of a physician commits fraud without the physician's knowledge, would the physician be held responsible?

Generally, a physician is considered responsible for the actions of his/her employees. But if the physician was not aware of the employee's fraudulent acts, prosecution would not be likely. However, the physician could be held responsible for any monies overpaid by the Medicare program.

Payment Policies

Admission for Observation

If our physician sees a patient in the office and later the same day admits the patient to observation at the hospital, would we be paid by Medicare for both visits?

No. Payment for an initial observation care code is for all the care rendered by the admitting physician on the date the patient was admitted to observation, per section 15504 of the Medicare Carriers Manual. This also corresponds to the AMA's CPT guidelines for observation care.

Billing Anesthesia

Are there differences between Medicare regulations and the rules of other third-party payers for billing anesthesia by the performing surgeon?

Medicare does not recognize modifier -47 (anesthesia by surgeon) and will not separately reimburse the surgeon for anesthesia administered by the performing physician. Other payers may allow separate reimbursement under the surgery code with modifier -47 attached, but payment across payers is inconsistent and some will not allow use of modifier -47. It is important to question your carriers about their policies when the performing physician administers anesthesia.

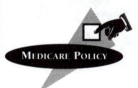
MEDICARE POLICY

Medicare does not recognize modifier -47 and will not separately reimburse the surgeon for anesthesia administered by the performing physician.

Quick Guide to Physician Fraud and Abuse Prevention

Charge Limits

Can physicians require patients to pay for services that physicians have never before billed for, such as telephone calls, prescription refills, and medical conferences with other professionals?

No. These services should not be billed separately. Medicare's policy is that telephone calls, prescription refills, and medical conferences with other professionals are included in the physician's visit or service, and that payment for the visit or service encompasses the payment for these items. If charges for such items come to the Medicare program's attention, they will be added to the charges for covered services in determining whether the physician has violated charge limits.

Colorectal Screening

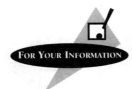

For Your Information

Colorectal screening, code G0105, is payable once every two years by Medicare for an individual older than 50 and entitled to Medicare Part B benefits.

How often does Medicare pay for colorectal screening for high-risk patients?

Colorectal screening, code G0105, is payable once every two years by Medicare for an individual older than 50 and entitled to Medicare Part B benefits. The Health Care Financing Administration (HCFA) considers the following diagnoses high risk:

1. Personal history of colorectal cancer

    V10.05 Personal history of malignant neoplasm of large intestine

    V10.06 Personal history of malignant neoplasm of rectum

2. Inflammatory bowel disease, including Crohn's and ulcerative colitis

    558.2 Toxic gastroenteritis and colitis

    558.9 Other and unspecified non-infectious gastroenteritis and colitis

    555.0 Regional enteritis of small intestine

    555.1 Regional enteritis of large intestine

    555.2 Regional enteritis of small intestine with large intestine

Payment Policies

555.9	Regional enteritis of unspecified site
556.0	Ulcerative (chronic) enterocolitis
556.1	Ulcerative (chronic) ileocolitis
556.2	Ulcerative (chronic) proctitis
556.3	Ulcerative (chronic) proctosigmoiditis
556.8	Other specified ulcerative colitis
556.9	Ulcerative colitis, unspecified

Diagnostic Tests

Are diagnostic tests payable under the physician fee schedule if performed by a physician assistant?

Yes. If the physician assistant is authorized under State law to perform the diagnostic test, it is payable under the physician fee schedule. Only a general level of supervision by the physician is required.

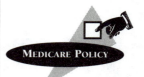

Medicare Policy

If the physician assistant is authorized under State law to perform the diagnostic test, it is payable under the physician fee schedule.

EGHP and Secondary Payer Rules

Could a situation exist where Medicare would not be secondary even if the patient has an employer group health plan (EGHP)?

Yes. For example, Medicare would the primary payer for a beneficiary with only Part B Medicare even if the patient is covered by an employer's health plan. This is based on Medicare regulations stating that a beneficiary must have both Part A and Part B Medicare for the MSP provisions to apply. However, it is uncommon for beneficiaries to have only Part B coverage.

Fee Schedule Data Base

What is the Medicare Fee Schedule Database?

This is a data file that contains information on services covered by the Medicare Physician Fee Schedule (MPFS). For more than 10,000 physician services, the file contains the associated relative value units, a fee schedule status indicator, and various payment policy indicators needed for

141

payment adjustment (e.g., payment of assistant-at-surgery services, team surgery, billable medical supplies, etc.).

"Free" Pneumococcal Pneumonia Vaccine (PPV) Shots

There has been some concern about the confusion caused by providers advertising PPV shots as "free." When patients later receive EOMBs, they contact the carrier to report fraudulent billing. Should providers advertise this as a free service?

Physicians, providers, and suppliers who accept assignment may advertise that there will be no charge for the PPV shots, but they should make it clear that a claim will be submitted to Medicare on the beneficiary's behalf.

Physicians, providers, and suppliers who do not accept assignment should never advertise the service as free since there will be an out-of-pocket expense for the beneficiary after Medicare has paid at 100 percent of the Medicare-allowed amount.

"Incident To" Defined

What is meant by "incident to"?

Incident to services and supplies are those furnished as an integral, although incidental, part of the physician's personal professional services in the course of diagnosis or treatment of an illness or injury. Auxiliary personnel performing these services must be employed by the physician or clinic and services must be performed under the direct supervision of the physician and billed by the physician.

DEFINITION

Incident to services and supplies are those furnished as an integral, although incidental, part of the physician's personal professional services in the course of diagnosis or treatment of an illness or injury.

Payment Policies

Modifier -22 and Payment

What are Medicare's payment guidelines for modifier -22?

Modifier -22, unusual procedural services, is appended to a code when the service(s) provided is greater than that usually required for the listed procedure.

Medicare guidelines concerning modifier -22 are as follows:

- Use modifier -22 to identify an increment of work that is infrequently encountered with a particular procedure and is not identified by another CPT code
- Modifier -22 can be used with all surgical procedures regardless of length of global period
- Use modifier -22 only with primary procedures, not secondary procedures identified with modifier -51
- Modifier -22 can be used for an assistant surgeon's services

Required documentation that should accompany the claim includes:

- A copy of the operative, radiology, or other applicable procedure reports
- A separate statement written by the physician clearly indicating the unusual amount of work in the case for the patient in question

Multiple Endoscopies

We can never figure out what we should be paid when more than one endoscopic procedure is performed at the same session. Are there guidelines for Medicare's payment policy on multiple endoscopies?

Medicare guidelines for multiple endoscopic procedures are based on the fact that all endoscopies include a diagnostic endoscopy. Endoscopies are grouped into families of codes, each of which includes a code for a diagnostic endoscopy (referred to as the "base" code). Since the relative value of

143

Quick Guide to Physician Fraud and Abuse Prevention

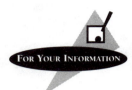

FOR YOUR INFORMATION

When both a base procedure and a related endoscopy with a higher value are reported, only the procedure with the higher value will be reimbursed since its value includes the base procedure value.

each endoscopy code includes the value of the base code, Medicare will reimburse the value of the diagnostic endoscopy only once. For instance, when both a base procedure and a related endoscopy with a higher value are reported, only the procedure with the higher value will be reimbursed since its value includes the base procedure value.

When multiple endoscopies from the same family and through the same body orifice are performed on the same day, Medicare will allow:

- The full fee schedule amount for the scope with the highest allowance
- A reduced amount for the additional endoscopies that is equal to the allowed amount of the additional procedure(s) minus the fee schedule allowance for the base procedure

The preceding guidelines do not apply when a physician performs two or more endoscopies from different families on the same day. For these services, the usual multiple surgery rules are applicable. This means Medicare will allow the full fee schedule amount for the scope with the highest allowance and 50 percent of the fee schedule amount for additional endoscopies of a separate family performed on the same day.

Three steps are necessary to calculate payment for multiple procedures from different families:

- First, multiple endoscopy rules must be applied to all procedures within each family. In each family, the code with the highest allowance is priced at 100 percent of its usual rate. Each additional code within the same family is priced at its fee schedule rate minus the allowable for the parent (base) procedure
- Secondly, the allowables calculated for all procedures in the same family are added together to come up with a total allowable for that family

Payment Policies

- Thirdly, the total allowables for the families are compared. The family with the highest total allowable is priced at 100 percent. Any remaining families are then priced at 50 percent of their total allowed amount

When a family of related endoscopies and an unrelated endoscopy are performed, the allowables for the related endoscopies are calculated first. They are added together to determine the total allowable for the family. Then the allowable for the family(s) is compared to the allowable for the unrelated endoscopy and standard multiple surgery rules applied. The higher allowable (family or unrelated procedure) is allowed at 100 percent of its fee schedule amount(s); the other is allowed at 50 percent.

For nonassigned claims, the limiting charge is 115 percent of the reduced amount.

No Set Fee

Can physicians bill for services that do not have a set fee and claim that no charge limits apply?

In such cases, physicians may have to bill an amount that they think is appropriate, subject to an understanding that they will roll back the charge, if required, to the Medicare charge limit determination. If no rollback to the Medicare charge limit as determined by Medicare is made, the physician is not acting in good faith.

Pneumococcal Pneumonia Vaccine

Does a physician have to be present when pneumococcal pneumonia vaccine (PPV) is administered?

Medicare does not require a physician to be present, but does require a standing order. However, the laws of some states may require a physician's presence.

Quick Guide to Physician Fraud and Abuse Prevention

Are a coinsurance amount and deductible required for the PPV benefit?

No. Medicare pays 100 percent of the Medicare approved charge or the submitted charge, whichever is lower. Neither the $100 annual deductible nor the 20 percent coinsurance apply. Therefore, if a beneficiary receives PPV from a physician, provider, or supplier who agrees to accept assignment (i.e., agrees to accept Medicare payment as payment in full), there is no cost to the beneficiary. If a beneficiary receives PPV from a physician, provider, or supplier who does not accept assignment, the physician may collect his/her usual charge.

Psychotherapy and E/M Codes

Can payment be received for psychotherapy provided on the same day as an E/M service or other psychotherapy services?

Under specific circumstances payment will be made. Payment will not be made for and E/M service the same day as individual psychotherapy. The physician work RVU for codes 90843-90845 includes the E/M work that would be provided to a patient on the day of a psychotherapy session. However, payment may be made for an E/M service the same day as group therapy (90847-90853) since the E/M services that would be included in individual psychotherapy could not be provided in a group session.

Payment will not be made for individual psychotherapy/psychoanalysis, codes 90843-90845, on the same day as interactive psychotherapy, code 90855. Group psychotherapy, code 90853, will not be reimbursed on the same day as interactive group psychotherapy, code 90857. Codes 90801 (psychiatric diagnostic interview) and 90820 (interactive psychiatric diagnostic interview) will not be paid on the same day.

Index

Abuse, 1-4, 6, 8-10, 12, 14, 16-20, 22-24, 26-28, 30-32, 34, 36, 38, 41-42, 44-46, 48, 50, 52, 54, 56-58, 60-62, 64, 66, 68, 70, 72, 74, 76, 80, 82, 84, 86, 88, 90, 94, 96, 98, 100, 102, 104, 106, 108, 110, 112-116, 118, 120, 122, 124-128, 130, 132, 134-136, 140, 142, 144, 146

Advanced Beneficiary Notification, 29

Anti-Fraud Provisions, 6

Anti-Kickback Statute, 4-5, 12-14, 37, 51, 112, 128, 136

Assistant Surgeon, 86, 143

Assumption Coding, 49, 79

Attorney-Client Privilege, 113

Balance Billing, 48, 50, 53-54, 131

Balanced Budget Act, 6, 36, 93, 112, 136

Balanced Budget Act, Of 1997, 6, 36, 136

Beneficiary Incentive Program, 12, 115

Care Plan Oversight, 56-57, 81-82

Certificates Of Medical Necessity, 4

Charge Limitation Amounts, 4

Charge Limits, 120, 140, 145

Checklist, 42, 47

Chiropractic Services, 93

Civil False Claims Act, 124, 133

Civil Investigative Demand, 115

Civil Monetary Penalties, 4-6, 8-9, 11, 16, 116-117, 120-122

CMN, 3

Cmps, 8, 18, 116

Colonoscopy, 86

Colorectal Screening, 140

Common Risk Areas, 48

Compliance Officer, 21, 23, 25, 30-31, 51, 113-114

Compliance Plan, 7, 11, 21, 23, 26-28, 30-31, 41, 48, 50, 52, 113-114, 135

Compliance Program Guidance Of Individual Practices, 20

Compliance Program Guidance Of Small Group Practices*****

Confidentiality, 25, 51

Conscious Sedation, 58-59

Consultations, 15, 81

Correct Coding Initiative, 16, 44, 57, 80

Corrective Action, 27, 44, 49

Cost And Risk Hmos, 32

Criminal False Claims Act, 124

Criminal False Statements Act, 124

Criminal Penalties, 4, 6, 10, 12

Critical Care Services, 49, 82-83

Cystourethroscopy, 83

Damages, 7, 9, 27, 54, 112, 116, 125, 129

Defrauding, 6

Department of Health and Human Services, 6, 19-20

Department of Justice, 8, 13, 18, 126

Diabetes, 95-96

Dietitian, 96

Disciplinary Action, 22, 26

Discount, 13-14

Documentation, 21, 24, 42-43, 45, 47-48, 51, 74-75, 79, 84, 88-90, 96, 120, 143

Duplicate Billing, 49-50

Education And Training Programs, 21, 24

Effective Lines Of Communication, 25

Employer Group Health Plan, 141

Exclusion, 4-5, 8, 10-11, 16, 18, 54, 62, 108, 112, 117-120, 122-123, 125, 127, 129, 135

Exclusions, 7, 10-11, 18, 29, 117

Explanation of Benefits, 44, 61

Federal Hospital Insurance Fund, 9

Federal Hospital Insurance Trust Fund, 6

Federal Sentencing Guidelines, 21, 28, 124

Financial Relationship, 5, 15-16, 33, 112

Fines, 6-7, 9, 12, 18, 31, 54, 112, 124, 127, 129

Fraud, 1-4, 6, 8-10, 12, 14, 16-20, 22-24, 26-28, 30-32, 34, 36, 38, 41-42, 44-46, 48, 50, 52, 54, 56-58, 60, 62, 64, 66, 68, 70, 72, 74, 76, 80, 82, 84, 86, 88, 90, 94, 96, 98, 100, 102, 104, 106, 108, 110, 112, 114-116, 118, 120, 122, 124-137, 140, 142, 144, 146

Fraud Alerts, 1, 9, 16-17

HCFA-1500 Claim, 30, 55, 57, 60, 62, 70-71, 73-74, 98

Health Care Financing Administration, 1, 19, 45, 125, 140

Health Care Fraud And Abuse Control Account, 6, 9

Health Insurance Portability And Accountability Act Of 1996, 1, 6, 54, 80, 116, 126

Healthcare Integrity And Protection Data Bank, 127

History, 3, 44-47, 88, 91, 121, 140

Hotline, 22, 25, 115

Incident To, 63-66, 96, 142

Initial Audit Report, 49

Injections, 66-67

Kickback, 3, 7, 13, 112

Knowingly And Willfully, 4, 6, 12-13, 54, 112

Legal Audit, 50

Liability, 2, 17, 29, 32, 59, 64, 66, 94, 100, 114, 123, 132

Limited Licensed Practitioners, 71, 96

Limiting Charges, 54, 60, 94, 131

Locum Tenens, 96-98

Mandatory Exclusions, 10

Medical Necessity, 3-4, 22, 49, 59-60, 74, 94, 96, 99-100, 108, 120-121, 129-130, 132

Medical Necessity Denials, 99

Medically Necessary, 2, 4, 6, 11, 22, 29-30, 59, 73-74, 94, 96, 99-100, 105, 111, 117-118, 120-121, 124, 130

Medicare Fee Schedule Database, 141

Medicare Integrity Program, 19

Medicare Secondary Payer, 34

Medicare Summary Notice, 115

Monetary Rewards, 12

Index

Monitoring Tools, 51

Most Favored Nation Clauses, 132

Multiple Endoscopies, 143-144

Mutually Exclusive, 80, 87

Noncompliance, 41-42, 71, 117

Noncovered Services, 4, 59, 96, 101-102

Noncovered Services, 4, 59, 96, 101-102

Nonparticipating Providers, 54, 70

Nonphysician Practitioner, 61, 66-67, 95

Non-Retaliation Policy, 25

Nurse Practitioner, 66, 87, 95

Nursing Facility Admissions, 73

Office Of Audit Services, 126

Office Of Civil Fraud And Administrative Adjudication, 126

Office Of Investigations, 126

Office of the Inspector General, 1, 8, 19-20, 45, 125

Omnibus Budget Reconciliation Act Of 1989, 5

Operation Restore Trust, 1, 18

Opt Out, 35-36

Opting Out Of Medicare, 36

Optometrists, 36, 103

Oral Medications, 67

Overpayment, 111

Pap Smears, 105

Peer Group Organizations, 125

Permissive Exclusions, 10-11

Quick Guide to Physician Fraud and Abuse Prevention

Physician Assistant, 66, 86, 95, 141

Physician Referral, 16, 106, 112

Pneumococcal Pneumonia Vaccine, 73, 105-107, 110, 142, 145

Postoperative Care, 73-74

Ppd Test, 86

Preventive Care, 59, 93

Price Reductions, 13-14

Professional Courtesy Discounts, 133

Prolonged Services, 75

Provider Self-Disclosure Protocol, 7

Qui Tam, 133

Rebate, 3, 13

Referral Prohibitions, 112

Referral Services, 55

Referrals, 4, 10, 15, 37-39, 108, 128-129

Remuneration, 13, 112, 117

Rental Space, 37

Safe Harbor, 5-6, 13, 39, 112

Sanctioned Individuals, 7, 22, 49

Self-Audits, 52

Self-Referral Prohibition, 15-16

Sentinel Node Biopsy, 89

Social Security Act, 10, 54, 62, 64, 104, 107, 112, 116-117

Special Advisory Bulletins, 18

Stand-By Services, 76

Standing Order, 105, 136, 145

Index

Stark Law, 5

State Medicaid Fraud Control Units, 125

Surgical Tray, 68-69

Telephone Calls, 54, 140

Third Party Billing Companies, 49

Treating Relatives, 108

Unbundling, 3, 16, 48-50, 57, 80, 90-91

Unbundling, 3, 16, 48-50, 57, 80, 90-91

Upcoding, 3, 48, 50

Violation, 5-6, 12-14, 26-27, 62, 112, 117-119, 130, 133

Waiver Of Liability, 29

Waste, 6, 8, 23-24, 31-32, 114-115, 125

Whistleblowers, 2, 22, 45